LIFE AFTER HEAD INJURY

JR JOSEPH ROWNTREE FOUNDATION

The Joseph Rowntree Foundation has supported this project as part of its programme of research and innovative development projects, which it hopes will be of value to policy makers and practitioners. The facts presented and views expressed in this report, however, are those of the authors and not necessarily those of the Foundation.

Life After Head Injury

The experiences of twenty young people and their families

JANE HUBERT

Department of Psychology, University of Southampton

Division of Psychiatry of Disability, St George's Hospital Medical School, London

with best wishes

Jane Hubert

Avebury

Aldershot • Brookfield USA • Hong Kong • Singapore • Sydney

Published by
Avebury
Ashgate Publishing Limited
Gower House
Croft Road
Aldershot
Hants GU11 3HR
England

Ashgate Publishing Company
Old Post Road
Brookfield
Vermont 05036
USA

British Library Cataloguing in Publication Data
Hubert, Jane
Life After Head Injury: Experiences of
Twenty Young People and Their Families
I. Title
362.19751

Library of Congress Catalog Card Number: 95-078094

ISBN 1 85972 148 6

Typeset by Cressida Fforde, Department of Archaeology, University of Southampton

Printed and bound by Athenæum Press Ltd.,
Gateshead, Tyne & Wear.

Contents

Acknowledgements

I am very grateful to the Joseph Rowntree Foundation for funding this research project, and to the members of my advisory group: Andy Alaszewski, Dorothy Atkinson, Barbara Lacey, Michael Oddy and Linda Ward, for their support and advicc. I would also likc to express my gratitude to Linda Ward for her unfailing patience, and for the interest and support that she has always given to my work. My heartfelt thanks also go to Peter Ucko for his encouragement and advice. Finally, my greatest debt is to the young people and their families who took part in the project and were prepared to relive a highly distressing period of their lives. I thank them for this, and for their time and hospitality.

Note

All names of individuals and families have been changed, and minor details altered throughout the text, in order to preserve anonymity. Members of those families which have been documented in the form of case histories have seen and approved the final text.

Introduction

Two years ago, riding his motorcycle home from work on a wet November evening, Jerry Cummins swerved to avoid a van that came out of a side turning without warning, and his motorcycle slipped into a long, uncontrollable skid. As the bike stopped dead against a lamp post, he was thrown forwards, hitting his head on the ground with such force that the side of his helmet was flattened by the impact. Within twenty minutes of the crash an ambulance was at the scene, which carried him unconscious to the nearest Accident and Emergency Unit. Jerry does not remember the accident, nor the hours or weeks that followed, but his parents do. Half an hour after Jerry had been taken to hospital, his mother opened the door to a policewoman who uttered the words that she had always dreaded: 'Your son has had a serious accident. I think you and your husband had better come to the hospital at once'. With what seemed to her later to be immense calm, Mrs Cummins rang her husband to tell him to come to the hospital, turned off the oven, left a note for her daughter, picked up her handbag and followed the policeman to the waiting car.

It was only when she got to the hospital and saw Jerry lying there as though dead, hooked up to machines, tubes, drips and monitors, that the full horror began to dawn on her, and then seemed to envelope her altogether as the doctor told her and her husband that it was unlikely that Jerry would live. This was the beginning of a month-long vigil beside their unconscious son, watching and waiting for signs of returning life.

What happened to Jerry is an every day occurrence. In Great Britain about fifteen people are taken into hospital every hour with a head injury and, every two hours, one of these will die (Torrens and Cummins n.d.). This book is about twenty young men and women who received severe head injuries but who did not die, although in almost every case it was not clear in the early stages, as with Jerry, whether they would survive or not. The aim of this in-depth study was to document the effects of severe head injury on family relationships, and the impact it has on the lives of the young people themselves, and on the members of their families.

The highest incidence of head injury is among people in their late teens and early twenties, and this study was restricted to people in this age group (from sixteen to twenty-five years old at the time of their injury). Three quarters were male, which reflects the predominance of young men in head injury incidents. The head injuries were mainly incurred in traffic accidents: seven in motor bike accidents, eight in cars, one on a bicycle, two as pedestrians. Only two injuries were not related to traffic accidents.

The families were first interviewed within eighteen months of their discharge from hospital (four within the first month) and were visited at intervals over the following year. Apart from age and length of time since leaving hospital, further criteria were that they should be unmarried, and currently living at home with at least one parent. Most of them had not left home before the accident, and none had yet established a supportive network away from home.

Twelve of the head injured people returned to live with both parents, five to a mother who had remarried or was living with a partner (though one young man almost immediately moved away to live with his father and father's partner); three lived with a divorced or widowed mother. Some of these family situations changed over the period of the two year study, and a few of the young people moved away from home altogether. This story, however, begins much earlier, before the head injured person is even aware of the event that is to have such a profound effect on his or her own life, and of all members of the family.

The suddenness and unexpectedness of a severe head injury means that for the families and friends there can be no preparation for what happens next, no planning of arrangements or strategies. There is, inevitably, only confusion, disruption, shock and despair. In these families, unlike those in which a baby is born ill or potentially disabled, there is an adult social being involved - an adult son or daughter. Until this moment they have lived a 'normal' life, growing up through childhood attracting just as much, or as little attention as any other young person, growing into adulthood gradually and comprehensively.

The first reactions are to the trauma of the accident itself. Individual shock and despair are often, at this stage, wrapped up in the group experience of the crisis, as friends and relatives gather round. There are tears, hugs, sympathy, helpfulness, and a disruption of the daily lives of all the people involved. The family has to cope with this crisis - react, respond, survive, almost live in the hospital and completely reorganize their daily routines.

They will discuss among themselves how it happened, whose fault it was, whether it was foreseeable, whether they could have prevented it. Was he or she drunk? Were the friends to blame? How could things have been different? Above all, will he or she live or die, and if they survive, what effect will this severe head injury have?

Although frequently used (including, for convenience, in the following pages), the term 'severe head injury' is not in fact a very useful term, especially in the context of a book that focuses on a period some months after the accident, because the outcome of head injuries, however similar they seem to be at the time, will vary widely. A head injury is generally categorized in the first instance by the use of the Glasgow Coma Scale, which is based on tests that assess the depth of coma in terms of motor and verbal responses, and eye opening. The score (from three to fourteen) reflects a range of severity, from a deep coma to mild confusion, and a score of seven and below is said to indicate 'severe head injury'. Another method of assessment that is also used, retrospectively, is the length of the period of time that someone cannot remember anything about, following the accident, but this too may not necessarily be a good indicator of what will happen in the future.

This book is based on a study that set out to document the effects that a severe brain injury has on an adolescent or young adult, in terms of their own social and familial relationships, and those of the other members of the family. It is not concerned with the physiological aspects of the injury, only with the effects that the injury, whatever its specific characteristics, has on the lives of the people involved. What happens when someone comes home from rehabilitation, to them and to their families? What sort of problems arise? Could these been avoided? Do members of the family get the advice and support that they need from the rehabilitation services? What happens to relationships within the family, and with friends? Is there anyone to talk to about problems and worries? What do the young people and their families feel that they need in terms of help, support or advice? These are the sorts of questions this study hoped to be able to answer.

The wide-ranging effects of severe head injury have been recognized by clinical and rehabilitation teams, but there is little detailed and qualitative material available to enable them to plan and provide effective services (including family counselling), so that the stresses that arise in families could be avoided or alleviated. The aim of this study was therefore not only to document the effects, both in the short and long term, on the family, but also to investigate the current availability of services to people who have suffered a severe head injury, both in the short and long term, and the sort of help and services that they themselves, and their families, feel that they *should* have.

Although much has been written about the physical, cognitive, psychiatric and behavioural problems arising from severe head injury, there is far less material relating to the familial and social circumstances that then arise, and most of this literature relates primarily to psychological rather than social factors (Brooks 1984; Lees 1988; Livingston 1987). From such material as there is it is apparent that head injury will have serious effects on the families concerned, in terms of their way of life, their needs, and their individual roles and relationships, both within the household and with the outside world.

The difficulties that arise for families are varied. Some arise from the fact that the head injury has caused some degree of change in the personality and way of behaving of the person with a head injury; there will also be problems for them, and for their parents, in adjusting to different, probably diminished, hopes and expectations for the future; there may also be a narrowing of social relationships and activities.

The attitudes, beliefs and emotions of members of the family - the injured people themselves, mothers, fathers, sisters and brothers - need to be better understood if services to families are to be effective. There is evidence that medical practitioners and other professionals may tend to be preoccupied with physical and cognitive improvement in their patients, and are less aware of the familial problems that may in fact be increasing at the same time (Lees 1988). The unexpected (by definition) occurrence of head injury presents the people themselves, and their families, with a totally unfamiliar situation, changing their way of life and social worlds and, in many cases, creating serious social and familial problems (Lezak 1978; Weddell, Oddy and Jenkins 1980).

Thus when people are considered well enough to go home, whether a few weeks or even over a year after the accident, the doctors and other members of the rehabilitation team may feel, often quite justly, that their patient has made remarkable progress. For the families this is the time when, quite literally, the implications and consequences of the head injury are fully brought home to them.

A serious injury of any kind will precipitate a crisis situation, creating anxiety and disruption to the lives of the family. But in the case of head injury there is more to the situation than just a physical injury. Head injury is also brain injury, and the brain controls almost everything - the ability to move, see, hear, feel, remember, think. Gradually families come to realize that in addition to the crisis itself, they face the possibility that their son or daughter will be changed in a number of ways, and to a greater or lesser extent - perhaps only for months, perhaps for a few years, perhaps for ever.

For most of the families in this study the problems that head injury brings with it are still very much in evidence, even for those in which the accident was over three years ago. Relationships within the household are still being renegotiated, the head injured young people are still being protected from harm as far as possible, and in many cases they are fighting against this protectiveness. For the people themselves there are problems of memory loss, inability to concentrate, of mood swings, violent emotions, insecurity, fear of being considered inferior or of being 'not all there', and so on. In most cases they have lost their pre-existing lives, their jobs and many of their friends. Every member of the family will experience the effects of all this, as well as having to deal with their own emotional reactions to the changed personality, and often lack of insight, of their head injured relative. Almost inevitably, it is the parents who struggle to keep not only their own lives going, but also the lives of all the other members of the family.

1 The hospital experience

The beginning of any story of severe head injury usually starts with a mystery. Often no one knows exactly what happened - the people who suffer the injury have no memory of the accident, nor of the moments, hours, days or sometimes months that led up to it. After the event, the head injured person will also be unaware of what is happening around him or her, or at least will probably be unable to recall anything. Thus it is the people around them - their parents, sisters and brothers, girlfriends and boyfriends who experience the initial anxieties and lack of certainties about the future. There is, to begin with, uncertainty about whether the young person will survive at all and, if they live, whether they will 'wake up' or remain in a 'persistent vegetative state'. If they do recover, will they be paralysed? Will they be in a wheelchair? Will they be able to speak, and so on - and, arising from all these questions, will we be able to manage him or her at home? What will happen to our lives? Will anything ever be the same again?

Immediately after the accident parents, brothers and sisters, and sometimes an assortment of friends and relatives set up a vigil by the bedside of the unconscious young person. Usually at least one parent would spend all day at the hospital, sometimes the night as well, often operating a shift system so that there would always be someone there. One of the hospitals, to which many of the young people were taken immediately after their head injury, provided a hostel for close relatives who lived at some distance from the hospital, so that they could be near the hospital at all hours of the night and day. The person who ran the hostel was highly praised by the families who stayed there, and the facilities were said to be 'absolutely superb'.

In most cases it was the mother who spent the longest time at the bedside, watching the machines and the drips and the monitors that were part of the 'life-saving' process. As time passed, the friends and relatives who initially shared in the watching and waiting tended to visit less and less frequently, and in some families one or both parents (or a parent and partner) were soon taking all the strain of visiting. Apart from the effects of this pattern of constant and prolonged visiting on life at home and on family relationships (see below), there were a few cases in which families endured considerable hardship in order to visit regularly. In the case of one family, hostel accommodation was not offered, presumably because they were considered to live near enough to the hospital to get there without difficulty. This would have been true if they had been able to afford public transport, or had access to a car, but this was not the case. As a result they walked for about an hour and a half every morning to the hospital, and again late at night to get home.

In some families it seems that very little help or advice was offered, or at least seen to be offered, even when direct appeals were made to service personnel, including social workers. A few families, for various, unconnected reasons, were already isolated from, and suspicious of official service organizations, and it appears that, even in such dire circumstances as these, the professionals did not succeed in establishing adequate communication with the families. Thus even when facilities were available for relatives, some families still slipped through the net, reinforcing the sense of isolation they already felt.

'You find the strength from somewhere'

In spite of the stress and anxiety in the days after the accident, when families look back at the acute stage in intensive care there is a strength and positiveness in what they say, and the way in which they say it, that is seldom apparent in the accounts of their current lives, now that their son or daughter is at home.

This is not to suggest that what happened to them was not seen and felt to be a catastrophic occurrence, even a tragedy; but many parents found reserves of strength that they had not known they possessed, a strength which enabled them - and their injured son or daughter - to get through the crisis period. As one mother put it 'You just keep going, you get this terrific energy from somewhere'. Another, whose son had suffered considerable facial injuries as well as a head injury, said:

> If I wasn't strong, I tell you what, I wouldn't be here today, no way, no way. I've had a long hard struggle. I mean, it was *hard*, and I had to be strong to keep *him* going, otherwise he wouldn't have.

One father, who suffered from chronic ill-health said: 'At the time you find the strength from somewhere to do it and you never ask yourself how long it can go on for'. Like many of the parents, he lived from one day to the next until his son came home, and then his energy ebbed away again and he felt that he would not have been able to carry on any longer.

Almost every parent was told, in the first hours or days, that their child might well die or, if not, would be in a persistent vegetative state - what they generally referred to as being a 'cabbage'. By definition, all the young people in the study survived. Looking back, many of the parents felt that they should have been given more hope at that stage, although at the same time they also wanted to be prepared for the worst. In fact, many of the young people were quite obviously very near to death at various times after the initial trauma. In one case the police even applied for the coroner's report: 'They didn't expect him to even get to hospital, and they told the driver of the other vehicle that he was dead' (and see below). In some instances a parent's belief that their child will live seems to be against all apparent odds. In fact it is less a belief that they will live, than a denial of the possibility that they will die. As one woman said, even when 'the vicar' came to administer the last rites, she refused to accept that her son was dying.

In order to survive the horrific circumstances in which they found themselves, many other parents also simply refused to accept the prognoses that were given to them during the first days or weeks following the accident. They argued with doctors, shouted at the nurses, and sat by the bedside for inordinate lengths of time, willing their son or daughter to wake up. The grim prognosis was often taken as a challenge, and this supports the suggestion from Brooks (1991) that the denial of the severity of the situation is a coping reaction, which may be very effective, at least in the short term. One mother graphically describes this:

> The doctor there told us that he would be better off dead and we ought to switch the machine off and let him die in dignity. I said 'no, just get out!' and he said 'he's only going to be a cabbage if he lives, you might as well let him die, you wouldn't want that'. And instead of being miserable, you know, saying 'well this is the end' or sort of start crying or praying or whatever people do, we just suddenly started kicking his arse and telling him to pull himself together, and that he'd gone through the worst of it, there was nothing wrong with him and he had no bodily injuries and we *shouted* at him. We didn't stop from quarter to seven in the morning until half past twelve at night.

Another mother, as she listened to the doctor telling them that their daughter was likely to die, said that she became totally focussed on the situation. She became 'tunnel-visioned' and the rest of the world became irrelevant: 'I was getting her back if it killed me. Whatever happened she was coming back'. Many parents reacted in a similar way, and were galvanized into a determined effort to bring their son or daughter back to life:

> All I did was pray, pray, pray: please just come out of it, come alive. I wanted him back - even if he was a cabbage that wouldn't have worried me as long as he was alive...I wanted him to be *alive*. I couldn't have handled it if anything had happened to him, no way could I have handled it.

One mother, whose son appeared to be making little progress in the early weeks, opposed the hospital's decision to move him into a local 'mental hospital':

> I was convinced he would come round...the doctor told me he would be a cabbage more or less. He said that they didn't think there'd be any hope for him, but I wouldn't let him go. I refused flatly, we sat on the bed when the ambulance came for him, we wouldn't let him go.

The refusal to believe that a son or daughter is going to die may be vented in anger not only towards the doctors who give the prognosis, but also towards the young people themselves:

> We were told by one doctor that he didn't think he was going to live. I flew at this doctor and said 'you've jolly well got to make him!' I don't know, somehow you just don't absorb it, you think, how dare they suggest such a thing, and you start getting angry then, because you know that your anger will sort of get things in order, and that's how it all seemed to come about. Because...I remember when I saw Phil for the first time I was so cross with him. I remember looking at him and thinking, fancy wasting somebody else's time like this.

The reality of the situation, that a son or daughter may be near to death, was often harder to grasp if there was no apparent external damage:

> He was laid out, plugged into all these machines, he looked like an angel, there wasn't a mark on him, and I couldn't understand what they were telling me. There they were telling me he could possibly die - and there was no blood, no cuts no breaks, no bruises. It was all in his head.

Parents varied in their reactions to the possibility that their child might survive but be what they called a 'cabbage'. Some, as seen above, wanted them to live whatever their condition, but others were less certain. One woman, whose son had been of exceptional intelligence, felt at one stage that it would be better if he did not survive, unless he could return to the intelligent, thinking being he had been before his accident. When she was told that he was likely to remain in a persistent vegetative state she said explicitly 'at that point I thought, yes, I *want* him to die then'. It is clear that some parents were very torn, not wanting to admit to themselves that they actually wanted their child to die, but not being able to envisage a future for them in a state of semi-existence. One father, although he does not say whether he thought at the time that his son should die, did say after the event:

> If somebody is going to be permanently damaged, brain-damaged for life, I'd rather they died, because they are not going to live a normal life again ever. You see people who are brain-damaged and it's a terrible state...they don't know what they are doing, they don't enjoy life, or anything.

Others expressed similar thoughts, and it may well be that more felt the same at the time, but were unable to express such emotions, even to each other, and later, when their children were recovering, were loath to admit to such feelings. Certainly some parents discussed it together, and the difficulties involved in talking about it are illustrated in this father's halting account:

> They didn't actually say that but the impression that I got was that he'd be a bloody vegetable...from being very, very positive - 'he's going to pull through' - you then get a kick in the you-know-wheres and you think, oh Christ, you know, if he does pull through what sort of standard of life is he going to have? One of the doctors said there was the likelihood of him being paralysed, couldn't speak - he really painted a very black picture...[my wife and I] spoke about it and I said, you know, they might actually come and ask us, you know, we might have to make a decision that - you know, do we want to keep the life support machine on, or off, you know, turn it off, or that sort of thing and I said, you know 'what do you feel about it?' And she just said straight away, 'I don't care what he's like, as long as we have him, even if he's a cabbage'. And I must admit I thought the same as well, I mean there's no way, as far as I'm concerned, that you could actually - I don't think that I'm as high a being as that, to make a decision whether somebody lives or dies.

In most instances the continuing improvement that parents saw in their head injured son or daughter when they started to return to consciousness pushed the thought of death out of their thoughts. Only one parent reports having doubts at a later stage of recovery in hospital. This was during a particularly distressing stage of recovery, when many of the young people became violent and abusive, and it is possible that other parents had similar reactions at this point, but were unable to voice them so explicitly:

> He was just swearing all the time and you couldn't get through to him...it was terrible, the language was so foul, and everything you tried to do for him he'd reject, and I kept thinking to myself 'oh, it would be so much easier for you if you'd have died. You wouldn't have had all this to fight', you know. It wasn't the fact that I was giving up, it was the fact that of everything that seemed to be happening to him there was no sort of *good* touching him anywhere.

Sometimes it was a long time - weeks or even months - before parents knew whether the pessimistic prognosis they had been given by the doctors at the beginning was correct or not. As they sat by the bedside they watched for signs of consciousness, waiting for their hand to be squeezed, encouraged and excited by the minutest movement that they believed to be voluntary - often in spite of the insistence by doctors or nurses that the movements were involuntary 'reflexes'. It was particularly hard for members of the family to sit by and watch their relative being moved about as though he or she was some sort of inanimate object. A few of them recalled the horror with which they witnessed their son or daughter being lifted from the bed and manoeuvred into a sitting position in a chair, still unconscious. Seeing them lying in bed as though asleep was one thing, but hoisted upright, in a mockery of normality, was terrifying. Some complained to staff, until they realized that this was being done for their own good:

> When [the occupational therapist] stood him up on this table and strapped him up, he just *hung*, and his mouth opened and all this dribble ran out, and I thought 'oh my God I've got a vegetable'...I was horrified, but they kept saying, 'no, he'll be fine, he'll be all right,' and I thought, you're telling me. When I went out that time I was gone, I had tears running down, I thought, Jesus, I can't handle this.

Nevertheless, she said she would have brought him home, whatever his condition: 'I wouldn't let anybody else have him because I don't think they could look after him like I could. Fiercely possessive of my own, I am'. Fortunately, she did not have to face bringing her son home as a 'vegetable' - he still has some problems, but he now walks and talks, and drives a car. As discussed above, although some parents thought that it would be better for someone to die than survive in a persistent vegetative state, all the parents said the same thing - that if their child had survived in this state they would have brought them home to live. As another woman put it: 'It's part of you, isn't it?' It is not possible to determine retrospectively what would actually have happened, and the fact that none of the young people in the study is now in a persistent vegetative state might simply mean that those who did not recover so well are in hospital, and thus were not included in the study.

However, there is no doubt that the intention was there when the possibility arose.

All the families praised the high standard of medical treatment received in the Accident and Emergency units and Intensive (or 'High') Care wards. The only criticism voiced by some was the lack of information about what was happening, and sometimes a dearth simply of anyone to talk to. Lees (1988: 166) suggests that 'hopeful but realistic facts' should be conveyed to families, and points out that there is an increasing body of knowledge about the outcome of specific injuries, which should be made accessible to relevant staff and to the families. In some cases parents said that they were given information right at the beginning, but they were too shocked to absorb it. Quite often they did not know who they should go to for information, or how the things they were told by different people fitted together. As Gronwall, Wrightson and Waddell (1990: 28) report, this can be a big problem, and they suggest that 'regular briefing sessions should be arranged so that the family knows exactly what is happening'.

In one case, the parents had constantly asked for information about the implications of the various stages their son appeared to be going through, but no one had seemed to be able to answer their questions. Much later, when they went into an office (in the rehabilitation unit) that they had not been in before, they discovered that the information they had wanted was readily available:

> There on the wall of the office it's got this chart of what you can expect of head injured people when they first come round, and what they do and what they do first, and this stage and that - very explicit. But at no stage of his recovery did anyone tell us any of it, neither during or now, did anyone say this is normal, this is what happens, it's followed by this, this is how it works. Nothing at all, and they know bloody well what was going on, it's all known, it's all known fact. And also I had the sort of vision that someone in a coma wakes up, you know, and smiles saying, 'hello mother' and gets up. Nobody tells you different. And they don't tell you that when the eyes open they're not going to *do* anything. So when his eyes opened I was thinking he was blind. It's so amazing, I am so stunned by how easy it would be to give people a sheet of paper - if you don't want to *tell* them give them a piece of paper.

Those parents who were allocated a specialist hospital social worker, or psychologist, when their son or daughter was taken into hospital, generally found them patient and helpful. Others, who had no one specifically named to talk to, tended to ask questions of any member of staff who would listen, thus getting a hotchpotch of individual opinions, as one parent pointed out:

> They didn't really fill us in all that much, it was more our inquisitiveness, and there were differences in what separate doctors said...invariably one would say one thing and one would say something else and, you know, you thought, Christ, what is going to happen? But they must have got absolutely sick to death of us because they kept saying to us, look, why don't you go?

In general, however, the actual work that went into keeping someone alive was described with unqualified praise and gratitude:

> This chap sat there at four o'clock in the morning telling me he was going to die - and he's alive! I'm grateful for that, I'm so grateful to the hospital and those wonderful nurses and what they did for him, you know. Well, there you go, you've got it, they saved his life.

During this crisis period parents learned a great deal of miscellaneous information and misinformation about brains and brain injuries in a very short space of time. Sometimes the sort of language used to describe an injury, presumably in an attempt to simplify the condition, conjured up distressing images; one parent was told, for example, that his son had 'burst his brain from the inside'. At the time, when parents are already in a state of extreme distress, such descriptions are not helpful. More careful explanations about the nature of the injury, and about the function of the various machines to which someone is connected, is more constructive, and may relieve some of the stress parents are under at this time, as described by one parent:

> I couldn't understand why my son had been going to die, and the person that actually explained that to me was [a psychologist]...she said that your skull is like a box with your brain in, and when it swells there's nowhere for it to go other than make your eyes sort of swell out a bit and of course it builds the pressure up down to the spine where the, is it the cerebellum, that's down here. And of course all the pressure, where it swells, pushes down...and stops the heart and stops the breathing, that's why he's on a breathing machine and they monitor the heart.

Apart from the galvanizing effect on parents that the depressing prognosis often has during the period of intensive care, as already documented, there is also another result. The fact that parents are told that their son or daughter may die, and that they are now, in almost every case, walking and talking, means that the early treatment may be seen not only as life-saving, which it very often is, but also in some way as having actually snatched their child back from death. This impression is enhanced by statements such as 'they said he died twice', 'we lost him', 'the police had him down as a goner', 'he stopped breathing' and 'they told us afterwards that he had died on Christmas Eve'. Thus, whatever happens later, this first stage of recovery is thought of almost as miraculous, and encourages parents to believe that their son or daughter is going to continue to improve at the same rate, and return to their former selves. As seen below, this optimism is often unrealistic.

So far in this account reference has been made chiefly to parents and other close relatives. In some cases there were others who felt that they were the ones who should be with the head injured person, and in a few instances tensions arose over who should actually be at the bedside.

In those cases in which the young person concerned had been in a relatively long term relationship with someone, that person assumed that they had certain rights, even that they had prior rights over the parents. Since the person with a head injury had no input into this debate, both parents and girlfriend (no boyfriends took on this role) could assume that it was their prior right to be at the bedside. In at least two cases this situation caused a serious rift between the families, which continued long after the boy had left hospital. In one instance, apart from the family feeling pushed to one side, part of the trouble was caused by the girlfriend's assumption that she had the right to carry out the personal tasks that needed to be done, and which the mother felt were her responsibility. The boy's father said he was made to feel 'like a stranger' in relation to his own son, and echoed his wife's feelings. Both parents felt that they had prior rights to their son.

This conflict also occurred in other families. Since the person with a head injury is not conscious it is, in effect, a battle over rights to his body, rights which the two families want to establish as their own before he wakes up and is able to make his own decisions. When this happens, the sensible acceptance by nursing staff that the head injured young man is an adult, and in an adult relationship with a woman, is sometimes difficult for the parental family to accept. They see their son as he is now, helpless and dependent, as he used to be as a child, and feel that it is their duty, or right, to care for him. In some cases they are right in their assumption that he is, or will be, their responsibility again, but meanwhile they find it difficult to step back and let him live the life he had chosen before, being cared for by someone else. In one family the tensions at the bedside resulted in a complete break between the two families. In this case the girlfriend's mother was said to have caused trouble between the two families, apparently resenting the boy's father visiting in the evenings. As a result, she is thought to be responsible for breaking up the relationship for good.

The tensions between the families of the young men and the families of the girlfriends might have been expected, since there is structurally almost bound to be a clash. The boys's parents consider that he is still part of their nuclear family, whether he had left home or not, and they revert to the parental caring role. On the other hand the girlfriend's family feel that at the time of the accident he was 'with her', and that this relationship overrides his familial ties. They are looking to the future, his parents to the past. In fact it proved each time to be the mother who, when it came to it, took on the responsibility of caring for her son when he left hospital, and, in the first case quoted above, handed him back to the girlfriend some eighteen months later.

The emotional tensions that build up at this time of crisis in the hospital can cause severe stresses within the family, quite apart from those with girlfriends and their families. In some cases the relationship between parents became strained during the early days or weeks at the hospital. One woman said 'we were like strangers' and another 'we just couldn't get close to each other'. Sometimes their ways of coping with their grief and anxiety were quite different, and this led to friction between them, making them prefer to be alone at the bedside. Almost all the parents (and their partners) in fact spent little time alone together at this stage, mainly because one or other of them was always at the hospital. Relationships with other relatives sometimes depended on their ability to control their own emotions; Mrs White, for example, when her mother burst into tears at the sight of her grandson in a coma, told her to leave: 'I said "get out! You are no good to me and you are no good to him"'.

The long, daily visits to the hospital often became a way of life, especially for mothers, and sometimes to the detriment of family life at home for younger sisters and brothers (and see Chapter Three). Quite apart from wanting to spend as much time as possible with their head-injured child, the ward routine, the nurses, the snatched meals in the cafeteria and so on, all became part of an increasingly familiar way of life. Life at home almost ceased to exist, and in a few cases a parent became quite dependent on life at the hospital, and found it difficult to stay away, as one mother describes:

> It got to the point when I couldn't stay at home, even if I knew someone else was going to be there, I couldn't stay at home - it was a way of life. We never ate here, all of us used to eat at the hospital - for five months I don't think I cooked more than a couple of meals here.

Another mother found that her life revolved round the hospital to such an extent that when her son was moved to another hospital, and she was discouraged from spending so much time with him, her life was suddenly quite empty:

> I felt, you know, 'Oh my God, what am I going to do?' It was just a way of life that completely changed you, to suddenly find yourself at home

again - I just felt lost and it was quite depressing, actually, being at home.

'He just seemed to be abandoned'

In many cases the move from the Intensive Care Unit, or a specialist neurosurgical ward, into a more general ward proved to be upsetting for the families of these young people. After days of close and intense monitoring following the accident, and sometimes one or more operations carried out in the first few days, the parents suddenly found themselves in an environment which appeared to pay little attention to their son or daughter, and sometimes staffed by people whom they felt had scant knowledge of head injury. In some cases the move was to an ENT (ear, nose and throat) ward, or to an orthopaedic ward or general surgical ward in the same hospital. For those families who lived outside the catchment area served by the hospital the move was often back to a local hospital, and occasionally parents tried to resist this move:

> They said they were going to move him to [another hospital] and I threw a wobbly because it's *miles* away, and also it was a back burner, [it] wouldn't offer anything, it's a geriatric ward. We were fighting it like crazy and in the end what they did, because we were obviously difficult parents, they transferred him without telling us; he was so distressed because he was conscious enough to know I wasn't around and he didn't know where he was going. He was three hours in an ambulance...and so when he arrived he was soiled, he went straight into an asthma attack - he couldn't breath, he was crying, he was hysterical, and so was I.

The very abrupt change in the level of care that was often apparent when the young people were moved, without reassurance from staff that this was a safe and acceptable state of affairs, made some parents distraught. In the words of one father: 'after intensive care it seemed almost neglect', and according to the sister of one of the young people: 'it was like another planet'. Many parents felt that the transition from intensive care to a general ward was too sudden, and the difference in care and attention too extreme:

> There was a total lack of care after he had come out of intensive care that morning, and we were absolutely frantic. They'd been taking temperatures and everything, every half an hour or so, and then - bang! It was about eight o'clock in the morning until teatime. It was dreadful - in fact we wanted to be there all the time, for protection for him...he was just laying there, they did nothing until about six o'clock at night...no

> drugs, no nothing, and he'd been on all this intensive care. He just seemed to be abandoned.

In some cases the perceived lack of communication between staff of the various wards, whether in the same hospital or not, and between staff and parents, was probably largely to blame for parents' uneasiness in the new situation. A communicative member of staff can transform the situation. This is highlighted by the reactions of one family, whose son was transferred to the same local hospital described above in such dire terms. In their case the presence of an informative and reassuring member of staff transformed the situation:

> They were exceptionally good to us, we couldn't have asked for any better support. He was in a coma for roughly two and a half months and the sister was more of a friend than anything, she was excellent, she really did tell us what to expect, all the stages he'd go through. She was absolutely fantastic and we can't praise the staff in that ward enough.

For this family, however, the euphoria did not last; the situation deteriorated when their son was moved into yet another hospital:

> That's where the trouble started. He was put into a ward with elderly stroke victims...the sister there didn't understand [head injury], never seen it before, and coming out of a coma he'd get very violent, it actually took five of us to hold him down one day. And, you know, trying to clean him up, because of his bodily functions - he'd got no control - the sister couldn't understand this, she didn't have a clue...he was in a terrible state, I went in and he had faeces on his hands and his face was covered...she said to him, and he was still in a coma, 'if that's what you want then you lay in it' and it broke my heart.

Other parents also complained that their children had been moved into wards full of elderly people, wards in which people were dying. In other instances, when the move was into specialist surgical wards, parents were concerned because their children seemed to be treated as though they were simple orthopaedic or ENT patients, whereas they had, in fact, recently suffered severe head injury. Because their primary concern was always for the safety and comfort of their own child, they watched closely and uncompromisingly for any error or carelessness on the part of medical and nursing staff. It can be argued that it is to the credit of these staff that they in almost every case accepted the presence, and the help, of family members. The criticisms levelled at them do not necessarily reflect the day to day, or hour to hour, care that was successfully given to these young people. However, there are obviously some occasions when the protectiveness of parents is in order, and there were understandable anxieties about the shortage of specialist staff necessary to cope with someone emerging from a coma, as one father illustrates:

> When he came out of neurological high care they put him into the surgical ward, which had never dealt with a head injury before. I found all broken glass beside the bed - he'd got out of bed with his drips and he pulled everything out and fallen. His arms were in a terrible state...he was thrashing around and they never had any bars up on the bed; he had sores on his elbows, his ankles were red raw; his catheter bag was just thrown on the floor under the bed and what made it worse was that he had a catheter infection, the tubes were full of blood.

This father was convinced that his son was thrashing around because he was in pain. In the intensive care ward he had been told that his son was likely to be in severe pain, but on this general ward the doctors only prescribed painkillers for him at night. When the doctor was tackled about this his attitude only antagonized the family further, and no attempt seemed to be made either to calm the parents down, or to explain why their son was behaving so violently, and on some occasions no nurse could be found on the ward at all.

It was only after some days of distress for these particular parents that their complaints were listened to, and then, as they said, their son got 'VIP treatment'. The father who made these complaints was backed up by his wife, but it should be said that he was hypercritical of the care received by his son, and some of his criticism reflects a general disenchantment with hospitals and hospital treatment. This is not to say that the level of care received by his son was necessarily satisfactory, but among the criticisms, and underlying much of what this unhappy father reports, is the lack of communication between him and the staff involved with his son. It is quite probable that they found him cantankerous and unsympathetic to their own problems of shortage of time and staff, but much unpleasantness might have been averted, in this and other instances, by overt acknowledgement of the distressed state that parents (and also other close relatives and friends) are quite obviously in, and realization that anger directed towards staff is often less a personal attack than part of a complex set of coping strategies.

Many parents reported incidents that had upset them: one parent complained that they found their son, who was disoriented and confused and had very bad sight, leaning over the side of the bed drinking his eye solution; a number of parents reported that their son or daughter had fallen out of bed, or repeatedly climbed out of bed and fallen on the floor; others reported that drugs, or eye drops, were not given as prescribed; wet (and occasionally soiled) beds were said not to have been changed promptly. On one occasion, when a drip had been wrongly adjusted, the father involved said: 'I thought, Christ, if we don't notice these things what the hell's going to happen?' His wife added: 'I told them straight: "when my son leaves this hospital I cannot say that he's had the best of attention. I'm absolutely disgusted".'

The role of parents was important throughout, and without them at the bedside it is probable that the return to normal functioning of some of these young people would have been slower. Certainly this is the view of some parents. When, for example, at a certain point, there was a choice between feeding through the stomach and through the mouth, then parents preferred to devote the time to the latter, rather than see their children 'full of tubes'. If possible they would feed their son or daughter themselves. One family, for example, sat with their son and fed him ice cream and jelly. His mother even bought chocolate bars, and: 'I bit it off in my mouth and let it melt and put it on his tongue and got it down that way'. In this way, slowly and painstakingly, they got their son to eat normally. His mother was convinced that, if they had not been there, the staff would have 'put all the drips all over him, fed him through his stomach and hoped for the best that he didn't pull anything out'. Whether this is what would have happened is not the point. What is important is that parents in this situation are not always given the information they need to properly judge the situation. Even though they have spent the last weeks or months in the ward, carrying out much of the care of their son or daughter, they tend to be treated, through lack of time or as a result of what they perceive as medical attitudes to ordinary people, as though they were incapable of understanding what was going on.

Another parent was concerned about her son's intake of food, because of his severe weight loss. Although it was being monitored, she felt that what was recorded did not reflect what he had actually eaten or drunk:

> He couldn't see, and he didn't coordinate properly, I'd gone in and he just had this whole heap of food in front of him...and he *did* drink, but he dribbled most of it, but they'd written on the chart that he'd had this, this and this. But everything was just down the front of him and on the floor...they weren't equipped to deal with his problems on that ward.

Looking back, parents can see that the constant battles they fought on behalf of their children probably appeared unimportant to other people. One mother, who had found it a slow and laborious business trying to get a beaker that her son could drink out of, said:

> These things sound so trivial now, but at the time, when you're in that position - it was extremely important to us and it was distressing, and I felt I never wanted to leave him.

In some instances injuries secondary to the head injury seemed to parents to be ignored for too long. Although they were aware that the condition of the brain was necessarily the first priority, some found the apparent lack of attention to other injuries upsetting. One family, for example, were worried about their son's eyes:

> Nobody had been round to examine his eyes, we were almost positive that there was going to be no sight in the right eye, but the left eye was very blurred. It was about three weeks after his first op before the eye surgeon came to see him and they discovered his eye was ulcerated, so they taped up the eyelid, the eye closed...and he was blind then, so he was totally disorientated and he wouldn't let anybody take the tape off because it would hurt, so we had a lot of behaviour problems with him then. And when he became allergic to the tape [the eye specialist] said, 'if we can't tape him up he's got to have these eye drops in hourly, it's imperative, it's got to stay moist.' I mean, try getting the nurses to do it hourly! It was a job getting them to do it four hourly let alone hourly, they used to forget completely.

Another family were anxious because nothing was done about their son's leg, although his other injuries, to his head and lungs, were being treated, and his life had been saved in spite of dire forecasts. By the time the leg was examined, after the parents had drawn attention to it, one toe was already gangrenous, and had to be amputated.

The perceived lack of attention to some of these young head injured people after the initial excellence of treatment was difficult for parents. They had weathered the initial shock and trauma, and the days of vigilance by the bedside, keeping an eye on the various machines that were keeping their child alive, and watching for any flicker of life. Now it seemed to them that their child was, as one parent put it 'on a back burner', and it was a battle to get the level of care that they felt was still necessary:

> We've never *been* in a position like this before, I've never had a serious accident or anything like that and it's an awful shock obviously, it caused us a lot of worry and distress. But on top of that, when you're fighting, you know, to get things that should be done automatically, *that* was what we found so upsetting and frustrating...then you start to find that nobody seemed to be able to tell you much about what was going on or what to expect...and there wasn't really anybody to talk to.

Often parents heard doctors talking among themselves at the bedside, but were not told anything directly, even though they were sitting there on the bed 'waiting on every word'.

The medical language used was not explained to them, thus however hard they listened, as one parent put it, they did not have 'the foggiest idea of what the hell they were talking about'. On the other hand, they did not want to be treated like idiots:

> For some reason they're *better* than anyone else in the world, and they're cleverer and they know more...and it's quite difficult to combat. They are still talking to me in a kind of Janet and John way, you know, as though they couldn't translate it into technical terms because I wouldn't understand it. They say things like 'well his brain goes round and round and round and something's gone wrong with it'.

Many of them would have liked to have someone to talk to about it all, right from the beginning, as suggested above, and to have had much more information. From the first hours in the Accident and Emergency Unit, and throughout the following months, many parents felt that they would have liked to talk to parents who had been through the same experience, someone who could say 'I know what you are feeling, I've been there myself'. In most cases the families were provided with a social worker, but this was usually to deal with practical issues, not to provide more general information and advice, or to act as a 'listener'.

For families who had struggled through the experience of having a son or daughter suffer a severe head injury, the accounts of major disasters in the national press were often greeted with some cynicism. It was remarked that considerable attention was paid to these major disasters, and that much time, effort and money was put into counselling for the survivors and their families. Why, some asked, should people involved in a major disaster attract so much professional help, when the individuals involved in single disasters tend not to be offered any counselling at all? In fact, these individual traumas may well be less easy to bear - there is no public sympathy, no public mourning, yet for each individual the pain and distress is at least as hard to bear, if not more so, since the experience is also a very lonely one. The contrast with large disasters is thus a very bitter one:

> How do these people who have these bad accidents up in London, you know, like the [Clapham] train thing, how do all these people get the counselling they get then? I mean why is it there for them? Is it because it's public and showy or what? For ordinary people it's happening every day...ordinary people are faced with it.

One of the 'grey areas' that parents would have liked to know more about was the question of medication. Although they accepted that sedating drugs were necessary during the initial days there were instances in which parents felt, in at least one case with the support of some members of staff, that the prescription of drugs was being prolonged for the convenience of staff rather than for the benefit of the patient:

> Every time he moved the girls were instructed to give him an injection to keep him still. You see he walked out of the hospital twice and he started getting a little bit active...it was all geriatrics in that ward and they couldn't concentrate on the rest of the ward and him as well. I went to see him one time and he was asleep all the time...even one of the girls said she was concerned that every time he moved more or less he was given an injection to keep still. Now that's when I started getting concerned about what medication he was on.

Whether or not the fears of this parent, and of others, had any foundation, it seems that no one thought to explain the situation in a way that might have relieved the anxiety that they were experiencing. There was, as one parent pointed out, a lack of counselling:

> Over at neurology I fully expected counselling for us, somewhere along the line, I actually said to the sister 'there's lots of things I want to ask, lots of things I need to know. Is there a counselling service or anything?' She said 'I'll get a doctor to talk to you', but we never saw anybody...we've had no counselling, nothing.

'They taught that boy everything again'

After the period of recovery in the post-intensive wards, whether specialist surgical or general medical wards, some of the young people were then moved again, some into specialist head-injury rehabilitation wards, others for rehabilitation in what were described as 'stroke wards'. Physiotherapists, occupational therapists, speech therapists and other professionals worked to return the young people to normal life. The general attitude towards their work was very positive:

> He was in there three months and those nurses...they taught him to use his waterworks, his bowels, to sit up, they taught him to walk, to balance...they taught that boy everything again, because he was a nothing.

Again, the determination of parents was evident. One mother, for example, when she was told that her son would never walk, and would be confined to a wheelchair, refused to take a wheelchair home:

I said 'he won't have that because he *will* walk'...we used to get him up on his feet: 'come on, come on, lad, *walk*.' And he did, in the end. He walked.

One parent criticized the rehabilitation offered to her son, not only because she felt it was wrong for him as an individual, but also because the philosophy behind it was flawed:

The difficulty is that he is a very individual person and he's an individual *adult*, he's not a child, and he's a very bright, intelligent person...and they're using childish materials. And that is so wrong, I mean we don't use childish materials when teaching adults literacy, we use adult materials. They have this sort of very unhappy habit of treating him like a half wit, and he now is saying 'why do I have to stay here? it's no good for me, it's not doing what I need' - and I know it's not what he needs; rehabilitation is an educational process, and to do it in the hospital makes it a therapy process; it means that people are ill, and you can't rehabilitate an ill person until you start to make them *not* ill. How do you rehabilitate in a hospital ward without institutionalizing? You can't, you have to move it to a more normal environment.

This was echoed by another parent, who resisted his son's move to a specialist head injury unit in a hospital some distance away, because he felt that life should be as normal as possible, not only for his injured son, but for the whole family.

For those who were having rehabilitation in a local unit, the transition from hospital to home was a gradual process. Time would be spent at the hospital and at home until the point came at which parents and staff felt that their children were better off at home, they were happier there, and benefited from the home environment and parental attention. Parents often said that such things as disturbed sleeping patterns and incontinence improved on the days that their son or daughter was at home - the latter said to be because parents were able to pick up signals better than staff in the hospital.

On the other hand a few of the young people would have preferred to stay longer in the rehabilitation unit. One said: 'It was like a family', and another: 'I didn't want to leave there really, I tried to stay up there a bit longer, it was good up there'. One interpretation of this could be that these young people had become institutionalized, but it should also be borne in mind that some of them were still very nervous and unsure of their ability to cope in the real world. In the hospital environment a clumsy hand, a slight limp, or unclear speech was just how they were, but in the outside world such things, however slight, would draw attention to them. Leaving hospital was the beginning of a life that would, for most of them, be very different from the one they had lived before.

2 The family: parental roles and relationships

When the young person first comes home from hospital, or the rehabilitation unit, the rest of the family receive him or her thankfully, but generally also rather cautiously. No one quite knows what it is going to be like, or how they should treat their relative after the experiences of the past months. The young people themselves tend to have their own problems to deal with, as described earlier, such things as memory loss, inability to concentrate for long, feelings of anger or aggression, mood swings, lack of confidence, physical difficulties, speech problems, and so on. These will affect them directly, and the people around them indirectly, especially parents (and see Chapter Three for the effect on siblings, and sibling relationships). There is a tendency for everyone to try very hard not to upset the person who has had a head injury, to avoid confrontations or outbursts of anger. Once this fear of upsetting someone becomes an accepted pattern it is hard to change it, and this can be an added problem (see below).

One of the hardest things for parents to deal with is the change in their child's personality. As one parent said:

> He is an entirely different person, it's just like having another son...no matter how many times you talk to him, it's still like meeting a new person each time...people say he's a nicer person now but I'd rather have him as he was before because, then, he was my son.

It is perhaps not surprising that the two families that appear to have had the least problems since their sons came home are those in which the young people concerned, although having severe physical injuries (to spine and leg respectively), are still very much the same in personality as they were before. Parents whose children are changed, however subtly, often go through a process of grieving for the child they have lost (Lees 1988), as one parent said: 'It does have all the hallmarks of grief'. The grief that is felt for the loss of an adult child may also be partly for the loss of a friend. One mother felt this very strongly:

> What I've lost is my friend. I've got a dependent son and I sometimes wonder what [the son that has gone] would make of it all, I sometimes wish he'd appear again so I could talk to him about it...its that loss, the bit that I would have gone to, to talk to about it - that's the bit that's gone...he's vulnerable, he's not mature, I couldn't lay my problems on him and I could have before.

One of the major problems in many of the families, especially in the beginning, is that the parents who have taken on the caring role - sometimes after a period without this responsibility - become very protective, but this protectiveness and anxiety for the safety and even for their son's or daughter's survival may appear to them to be unnecessary restrictiveness. Often it is hard for parents and children to agree in these circumstances, especially over such things as staying out late at night, drinking alcohol or taking drugs. These may be activities that parents and their children have fought over in the past, thus the current conflict may be intensified by the young people's awareness that they are again being treated as though they are too young to make their own decisions about they way they live their lives.

Although parents may be restrictive in certain ways, they may also be over-indulgent in other ways. When someone first comes home from hospital there is, quite understandably, a tendency to treat them preferentially, even as a special kind of 'invalid'. Also, since the young person usually tends to be easily upset, members of the family try to avoid situations that will cause trouble - the phrase 'walking on eggshells' is often used by the parents concerned. If this situation goes on indefinitely the person with a head injury becomes the controlling force in the household, and the balance of power within the family cannot return to normal. The power that the young head injured person has in these circumstances does not feel like power to him or her; they too feel powerless, as well as frustrated and angry.

Parents, too, may well feel frustrated and angry that their own lives, which many had recently begun to reclaim for themselves as their children left home, are again dominated by the needs of a dependent son or daughter (and see Gronwall, Wrightson and Waddell 1990).

Anger and frustration: 'Its a hell of a flaming trauma'

In the summer of 1991, twenty-one year old Glenn Carter was thrown from his motor bike and suffered a severe head injury. Because it happened on a

Greek island, where Glenn was working, his parents - not knowing whether they would ever see him alive again - set about collecting enough money together to fly to Athens immediately. When they got there, the nightmare of the next few weeks was intensified by the fact that it was taking place in a foreign country, among strangers whose language they could neither speak nor understand.

As soon as Glenn was considered well enough, he was flown back to England by air ambulance and later, after four months in hospital, he went home to live with his parents. By the time of the first interview with him, fourteen months after his injury, the situation in the household was extremely tense, and tempers quickly became frayed. The main problem, from Glenn's point of view, was that his family now treated him - and talked about him - as though he had become, in his words, 'a cripple'. From his mother's point of view the worst thing was Glenn's constant anger and frustration, vented mainly against her:

> I'm in the doghouse and I don't really know why. He comes out with accusations every so often which I find quite distressing because they're not true. There have been certain items which doctors have said to look out for, which I've been made aware of...and now Glenn's taken them as accusations. It doesn't matter whether I do right or wrong I'm afraid I'm never right...I'm not allowed to say anything in defence because I'm automatically stopped. I can never even explain myself, which is very frustrating. Glenn feels frustrated, but he never even accepts or realizes how I feel, because I'm never even allowed to speak, it's always through a third person.

Mrs Carter expresses something that many other parents feel - that they are expected to be understanding and endure ill temper and abuse from their son or daughter, but be endlessly patient and calm themselves. At the same time they have to impose restrictions on their children's activities, based on what they were told by the doctors, and these are often resented. Almost always, these parents are operating on a ragbag of odd bits of information culled from various different professionals, usually at an early stage. They do not know whether what they were told a year ago is still relevant or not, nor whether the labels that were stuck on then still apply, or in fact ever did apply, or what they actually mean. For example, one of the things Glenn Carter most dislikes is being called 'brain-damaged'. He insists that he is not, and it is very important to him that he does not have this label. His mother, however, says: 'It *is* brain damage, Glenn, it doesn't matter which way you look at it'. Glenn replies:

> It's *bruising*, it's not permanent damage...I know you love to refer to it as brain damage, like, 'my poor little brain-damaged son' - everyone thinks 'poor little brain-damaged Glenn'; basically you've said 'Glenn you're a brain-damaged cripple.' You have, why do you deny it? You know you have,so why deny it?

Neither Glenn nor his parents know what 'brain-damaged' means, and this is true in many of the families. For Glenn, the label implies something irreversible - he says that if he had another head injury and got brain damage, 'I don't want to be woken up, because I see those people in wheelchairs, like, dribbling away, if I end up like that that is worse than dying'. For the people who used it in the hospital, however, it seemed to be used as a shorthand term which could cover a wide range of conditions from bruising to permanent destruction of parts of the brain tissue. Thus Mrs Carter defends herself: 'they told me he had brain damage, every doctor, every nurse that we've spoken to has classified it as brain damage'.

When Glenn came out of hospital he was told to do certain exercises to improve his left side, which was slightly paralysed, and to use his left hand as much as possible. Glenn resents the fact that his parents tried to make him follow these instructions, because, to him, this implies acceptance of the 'brain-damaged' label:

> You said, 'Glenn, why aren't you eating your peas with your left hand' as if I couldn't! I knew I could, but I was eating, not performing a task. It really pisses me off, Dad was the same...I didn't do my exercises but it got better on its own. Which means it's not like permanent brain damage. I've got to wait for my brain to repair, haven't I, to let the bruising go away. That's when it gets better, when the bruising's gone away.

Some months after this conversation, Glenn was in fact told by the specialist at the rehabilitation unit that he had a 'bruise' on his brain, not 'permanent brain damage', and this made an enormous difference to him:

> I've now got a brighter outlook on life, and a new confidence because he didn't say, 'Glenn you've got brain damage you can't lead a normal life ever again' like you [his mother] always seem to say...he said I've got bruising to my brain, my nerves aren't damaged, they aren't killed and wiped out, they're a bit twisted and stuff, and that will come back on it's own.

In spite of Glenn's 'brighter outlook' he remained very angry at the world in general, and his family in particular. His mother tried to get a counsellor, when Glenn's anger seemed unmanageable, but so far she had had no response from the hospital:

> I think he needs counselling, I think he's bloody angry. I think he's damned angry. It really, really gets to me that he is just left to get on with it, you know, I mean yes it's fine for the doctors to say he's doing exceptionally well and boost his morale that way, but he really needs to get a lot of things out of his system and he can't say those things to me. It would be lovely if he could, but he needs practical help, not sympathy, you know. I think he's angry, he's frustrated, he's impatient. He really needs to get all of that out of his system, so it would help him to cope...it wasn't too bad when we had the [hospital] social worker who used to come round, she could help him get a few things out of his system, but she left.

When she stopped coming no one else came to talk to any of them. Glenn says 'I don't *need* a social worker'. When his mother mentions counselling Glenn argues that it would not make any difference anyway. One of the things that most upset Glenn was that his hair had been cut off, and from his point of view, however many times people say to him 'Glenn, your hair is quite long' it does not alter the fact that in his terms it is very short. Counsellors, he says, are for gullible people; they cannot alter the facts. Glenn is quite clear about what he needs:

> My counselling can be getting my bike on the road. If I've got my bike then I'm fine, that's all I need, my bike. I can't really explain that, *you* can't really understand that, but, like, I say to the doctors 'If I could ride my bike off-road that would sort me out'. And they say, no, it won't, going over bumps on a motorbike, that won't do you any good, but it will...they can't accept the fact.

It is tempting to believe him. Certainly on the days that he is going out to do something his mother notices the difference in him, and he feels much better (and this is also reported by other young people in the study):

> Like when I'm sat around the house, when I get up late, and I lay in, and stuff, just sit around the house doing nothing, just being lazy, I do feel, you know, sluggish or whatever. If I'm up early and I'm doing stuff, I'm fine.

Part of his frustration is because he knows he is vulnerable; he is dependent on his parents to house and care for him and to drive him around, but he desperately wants to be able to be independent again. The symbol of his independence is his motor bike, which he is getting into working order. He feels that when he can ride his bike again things will change. To him, as he says, his motor bike means 'freedom'.

Neither Glenn nor his parents really know what he should or should not be doing. At first, when Glenn was still in hospital, it was possible to ask questions, although his parents say that the answers often contradicted one another. But since he has been home, and the hospital has discharged him, there appears to be nothing in its place, as his mother says:

> This has been the problem all the way through, nobody has really been available for you to go and ask direct questions to - because you *want* questions answered, and you don't always see the right one, so you don't always get the right information.

Because of the different information from different people at various times, Glenn's mother takes the most cautious line, and Glenn the least. For example, one neurologist said: 'one beer and you are going to have a fit'. From then on Mrs Carter has lived in terror of Glenn having a fit: 'they put all these fears in your mind...I mean it's a terrifying thought'. Glenn, on the other hand, has tended to take no notice, and frequently went to the pub and got blind drunk. There seemed to be no continuing source of sensible advice, as Mrs Carter points out:

> They gave us such a lot of pep talks at first, on what we had to tell him not to do. I mean they put a lot of onus on us and that has caused a lot of bad feeling between us because I get over worried...after what he's just gone through, I mean, God almighty, it's a hell of a flaming trauma, and you think, flippin' heck; nobody else has come along...it is very, very difficult to know how to deal with everything all of the time, for Glenn and for us, we've never had any real back up. Nobody's ever even given us a book, you know, just to give you a brief explanation of the possibilities - the good possibilities as well as the bad; nobody's ever been at hand.

Glenn says that his mother is trying to keep him as an invalid, even though he is better, because she just enjoys looking after people. 'She wants me to be brain-damaged' he says 'because she always wants to look after something, like she's happy if the dog's sick so she can look after it...she likes to take it to the vet and pamper it and stuff'. His mother denies it, and tries to explain how difficult it has been to know how much to try and control him:

> He's too old for me to take control and say this is good for you and that's not good for you, and he's too young to really *understand* - he still doesn't appreciate the care, the upset, the whole worrying episode; he doesn't realize, he relates it to mummy being overprotective. I'm not being *over*protective, I am protective because I'm his mother, I can't

alter that. When he was in that hospital...I was plunged back into the protectiveness of real maternal instincts, and I had to kind of ease off, as he became more and more aware.

Glenn complains that his mother is still 'holding my hand when I go for an appointment'. She admits that she did at first: 'yes, I used to take you in as if you were a youngster, that's true' she admits. The trouble in this situation is that although in some ways Glenn was a 'youngster' again, in most ways he was quite clearly still an adult, and expected to be treated like one. His mother realized this, but could not help being concerned when, for example, he stayed away all night without telling her. Her dilemma was, and still is, that although she wants him to become independent, even to move out of the house, she also worries the whole time when he is out of sight. Glenn complained that on one occasion she rang the police when he was away for a few days. He says she treats him as though he is four years old, and that she had never rung the police when he stayed out before he had his accident. His mother says there is a 'slight difference' now, to which he sarcastically answers: 'Well, according to you, I'm brain-damaged now'. She replies:

> You were injured, and you just disappeared...you had an accident a year ago and you suddenly disappear for three days and two nights without a single phone call, yes I was bloody worried and if you expect me not to be - tough!

Glenn's mother had also been very worried about his drinking, and his use of 'speed' to get over his nervousness. She had told him that it was 'not advisable'. Glenn retorts:

> I didn't give a *shit* if it was advisable or not. I just wanted to get back to normal. I didn't care *what* I took. You don't realize that that's the thing.

Glenn feels that no one listens to him, that his parents will only look at the problems from their point of view. They try to restrict what he does, he believes, because they seem to think that he does not care about himself, which he says is wrong:

> I do care about myself a lot, no one realizes. They think 'Glenn's a drug addict, he likes to mess himself up' which is crap; you've got to realize that I didn't really enjoy myself over the last two years, I'm not exactly going to do the same thing again, am I?

There have been times when he has felt suicidal, and he says he has tried to explain to his family how he feels: 'But what's the point? No one listens. Do you listen?' he asks his mother, who replies:

I do listen when you speak to me and not shout at me, if you keep shouting and raging I'm afraid I just have to stop and go away. I'll talk to you any time you want to talk but I won't stand there and be raged at because it makes you feel better. I try to be extremely helpful wherever I can but that's not always appreciated. I mean the fact that *I* can get angry doesn't come into it, you talk to me like dirt when you're in the mood and in the next breath it's 'mum could you take me here...mum could you loan me a tenner, mum could you come and fetch me.'

When Glenn uses threatening language, and says he feels like smashing the place up, or punching someone, his mother says:

If you start doing that you'll definitely have to move out because I'm not having violence in the home. This is our house and you live by our rules, when you're under this roof that's the way it goes, that's the rules...don't live here if you feel like that" .

Glenn says angrily: 'I'd *love* to live somewhere else'. Both mean what they say, at one level, but at another level both know that at the moment they are stuck with each other. Glenn needs his family, but resents them and the care that they give, and what he perceives as a certain smugness - as he says cuttingly to his mother: 'You think you are Florence Nightingale, a saviour'. To her, having spent the last year devoting herself almost entirely to her son, this seems unfair:

Then in turn I can say I don't see why I should be bothered to go on when all I take is a load of stick for it. Why should I care if you don't care? If you don't care about me...I'll just get on with my life.

But she cannot get on with her own life, and she continues to worry about Glenn, because for all his bravado, she knows he is scared and lonely. When he insists that he feels fine, that he is not depressed, and should be allowed to do what he likes, she says - proving that she *has* 'listened':

Who turned round to me not long ago and said you actually thought of doing away with yourself? And I'm not supposed to worry? And I'm not supposed to interfere?

From the beginning, Mr Carter had been a great support to his wife; he was 'always there in the background, and he gave full support to us all, emotionally and financially'. In spite of this, the trauma of the head injury and its aftermath had a devastating effect Mrs Carter. The uncertainties, rows and lack of someone to turn to made her physically ill and depressed. About sixteen months after the accident, she went to see her GP:

> He actually put it down to just total stress. I felt as if I was going to have heart trouble, I was getting this shortness of breath, I kept having all these terrible sweats day and night. I was feeling really, really uptight and near to tears and near to anger, everything was too much, and I was flying off the handle.

Her GP put her on antidepressants and found her a counsellor, which she did find helpful, but she felt that it would have been much more help if it had been with someone who had some knowledge about head injury and the effects that it has. Even Glenn might have succumbed to pressure to have counselling under these circumstances, and the relationship between him and his mother might have been eased at an early stage in the recovery process. As it was, the process was very slow. Two and a half years after the accident Glenn is still at home, though relationships within the family have improved considerably. Glenn's reactions to his mother's 'motherliness' are less angry - when she answered a question that had been put to him he said sharply, but not angrily:

> You're doing it again, mum, taking over again. I am not slow, I can speak for myself, and I can think for myself. I'm not hard of thinking, I'm a bit hard of speaking but I'm not hard of thinking.

In fact that sums up his predicament very well, and he says that people should be told that a head injury does not mean you end up slow and stupid. 'That's what you should put in your book' he says 'people need educating'.

Mood swings: 'You're on tenterhooks all the time'

Unlike the Carters, the White family did have the advantage of someone to give advice and moral support from the time that Colin was in hospital. The Care Manager from the hospital was still visiting the family, albeit less frequently, almost three years after the accident, and would probably continue to do so. This regular visit was invaluable, and kept Mrs White going through some very hard times. However, it is interesting that when friends said to her that she should see a counsellor, she rejected the whole idea - she thought that it was better to just get on with things herself, not spend time telling someone about her problems. To her, the Care Manager, Jan, was not an official 'counsellor', she was someone who came to the house to talk and listen to Colin, and to them. She had become, in fact, a friend, but a friend who had a wide experience of head injury and its effects on individuals and families.

Mrs White, at each crisis point after the head injury, somehow found herself taken by surprise. It was as though she had to stay firmly in the present, otherwise things might become too difficult to deal with. One early example of this was soon after Colin came out of his coma. When his mother came to visit him the nurse said to Colin:

> 'Show mum what you can do' and...he went to get out of bed and I thought, why's he taking so long to get out and she said 'look, he can do two steps' and I thought, stupid girl, of course he can do two steps, and then they told me that he had to learn to walk... nobody had told me he couldn't walk, I suppose people thought that that would stand to reason. I thought 'you've got to learn to walk, I don't believe this', and I felt as if I'd gone off and dreamed. I mean, I had been sat in the hospital with him all the time and I just couldn't take it in that he had to learn to walk again.

Mrs White in fact puts into a nutshell what happens to almost every parent in this situation. From the moment of their child's head injury they are plunged into unknown territory, often confused and bewildered, usually with no one to guide them through it. At the beginning this is compounded by the sense of shock:

> You're not in this world anyway, you're in such a state of shock. You become automated, in your thoughts and in your actions. I think it's a bit because you're not in control and everybody else seems in control...And you see all this going on and it's just like as if you're in an inner play and you're there waiting for your part, it's really strange.

Colin finally came home, nine months after his accident, after a spell in a residential rehabilitation unit. At home, he attended a local day centre, and a sheltered workshop, for people with physical disabilities. By the time interviews with the family had come to an end, the White household was still very much dominated by its effects. Colin's own perceptions of the situation could not be gauged, because he was one of two young people in the study who preferred not to be interviewed. At the beginning of the first interview with his parents they denied that he was much changed from how he had been before the head injury. 'He's more or less how he was before' Mrs White said, and her husband agreed: 'He's just a little shorter tempered I think'. However it soon became apparent that Colin was in fact very changed:

> He's meaner, he doesn't seem to have so much sympathy as he had before for other people...he seems to think well, if you choose to get upset it's up to you, if you want to make a fool of yourself, he's hard like

that now...You don't expect rewards, I mean you automatically nurse somebody and care for somebody... but as he sees it, 'oh well if people want to waste their time it's up to them,' I think it's because he's got no confidence in himself at the moment.

But it is not only Colin's behaviour that has changed; to his mother it is as though he is a different person, someone she will never be able to know in the same way as she knew the son she had before:

> It's like the Colin we had has died, and although it's still Colin, it must be similar to when you adopt a child - I've got the same person who I gave birth to, but that person's developed into somebody that I don't know as well as I'd like to. That's how you must feel when you've got somebody else's child, that you want to know what's going on inside them but you will never know fully.

Like Glenn Carter, Colin resents the fact that his parents restrict his life: 'He seems to think we're living his life, and not letting him live it'. Colin also sometimes tries to blame his mother for what happened to him - a head injury which resulted from an action that could have been intentional, or not. Either way, it angers his mother to have this put on to her shoulders:

> I often get this outburst, 'it's all your fault. It's all your fault this has gone wrong in my life...all this that has happened to me is all your fault.' And you know it makes me cross, I say to him '*what* is my fault?'...'Well, if you hadn't expected so much out of me I wouldn't have gone, you know, gone and...' - he never says 'I wouldn't have gone and done it', but he always refers to the fact that part of him knows what he was doing.

Neither of his parents feel they are to blame, though Colin's father did feel at an early stage, and only briefly, that it must somehow have been his fault. Many parents say that they start soul-searching, and discussing with each other what might or might not have prevented the accident happening. At this stage they need somebody else to talk to, who would recognize these emotions and be able to talk them through with them. The Whites did have someone to talk to, but with regard to guilt, Colin's mother had been very definite from the beginning:

> I think he could have stood back and realized how fortunate he was to have a nice family...initially I felt very cross with Colin, and I do sometimes get cross with him now.

Mrs White gave up her job to look after Colin, because although he was out for most of the day she found that she could not concentrate on her work:

'I felt like I was going mad. I couldn't stand the pressure of Colin *and* work'. It is his anger and mood swings that are the most difficult to cope with. The doctor told them that it is just 'part of the damage', but his mother does not find this particularly helpful:

> You can't keep hiding behind the fact that it's the 'damage' because you've got to try and be one jump ahead of him all the time, because he'll be behaving like a normal teenage person, but suddenly it's like a mask will slip and the damage shows through so you've got to be one jump ahead of the thoughts. It is very difficult...one day he could be perfectly calm, more like before anything ever happened at all, and you just gear yourself to the fact that he's beginning to be what I call reasonable and nice and your whole system starts sort of unwinding, and suddenly you've got this angry person there again, and it happens when you're not looking - but I won't accept that I'm back to square one, I move half a pace along each time, because if I say, 'oh I'm right back' I find the whole of me sliding down again.

Sometimes she feels that 'its like you're in a sort of well and you can't climb up the side'. Their life is largely dominated by Colin's moods:

> Even when he's on a good run I've geared myself that any minute this might end, because you don't really know. It's the only way you can cope with it really, it's a bit of a strain, I must admit, because you've got to get on with life and you've got to cope with everything else that comes, daily events, and if he's on a sort of down run, somewhere along the line you feel, inside of you, the 'coping' person in you is becoming small. I can't describe it any other way, but the inner you is slowly shrinking, and if it gets any smaller, you really don't know how you'll cope...you dare not let go completely.

The strain is greater because she feels that she must not let her own moods become visible to her son:

> If you're a bit low yourself you tend to feel that you're letting the person down that needs your help because if you're not feeling strong that strength isn't showing to the person, so therefore they're not having as much boost as they should be having, because I'm sure the person picks the vibes up, and thinks 'oh, this is a vulnerable time' - you have really got to be one jump ahead.

Five months later (eighteen months after the head injury) things seemed to be getting better. They still had to be careful with him but he appeared to be getting 'back to normal'. Mrs White said it was like going back over the teenage years again: "you've got to repeat it all again'. Colin even talked of moving out, but decided to stay at home for the moment. His mother had mixed feelings:

> In some respects I'm glad he's been able to stand back and say, I have got a good home and I am better off at home at the moment, but there's another part of me that would like to see him move away. I don't mean move away and not bother to come back, but just move away, be able to be a little bit more independent.

Altogether they were all getting more settled, but a month or so later things had got much worse again; Colin was rude and aggressive at home:

> It's been *awful*, and the thing is, up to that point I suppose we got lulled into a false sense of security; I really couldn't believe how well everything was going...overlooking the fact that Colin still has a lot of emotional problems, so that's something that you've really got to sort of home in on. You learn a lot of things out of all this, you really do. But that's another point that people need to be made aware of...it's just so sad isn't it - I *can't say* that next month everything's going to be different and we can go down another course, because it's just not going to be like that is it? It doesn't matter what you're trying to do, I think all through the rest of the days of all the family, everybody's days are going to be affected.

Colin had become very threatening; he had punched his brother and even raised his fists at his mother, but did not hit her. Again she had this feeling that she was going to disappear:

> He said 'you're not ruling my life, I'm going where I want, you always want me to do what you want'...he gets like this, when he can't have his own way he just goes off in a sort of paddy, you know, I think to myself, well I'm not going to put up with this, it's not fair...and I just stood there and I mean Colin's quite tall now and I just sort of felt like I was shrinking, really actually physically shrinking, I was just so drained of what to say to him, I looked at him and I wasn't angry but I thought, what can I say that is going to have an effect, and the harder I was trying to think that, the more I felt as if I was shrinking.

Colin's father gets very upset by Colin's behaviour, and far angrier with him than his mother gets:

> Fred came home and I was telling him - he was stood out in the garden and his hands were going into fists, you know, where he was cross and he said to me, 'I shouldn't say it, Mary, but it would have been better if he'd died', and I said 'but he didn't and he hasn't, and it's something

we've got to live with, and you'll have to get used to it.' I was talking to him like I was talking to Colin, you know. And I thought, I've got two babies in this house, not one.

Although it is not obvious when Mr White is talking, his wife thinks that it has been more difficult for him than for her, in some ways:

> It hurts being a mother but to be a father and it's your son, I think that must hurt a man greatly...sometimes he'll say, 'if he'd have been much worse it would have been better if he hadn't been here' And then other times he'll say, 'you know, I really don't believe the recovery he's made'. I think he's very disappointed, I think he sees no end to it all, I mean I suppose as a mother you sort of feel it but you pretend, don't you, as a mother. I suppose it's a sort of big let down...it's very difficult to say, but I think a man doesn't want to think that there's anything wrong with his son, I think it's doubly hard for a man; Fred's had all these sort of hopes obviously, for him, like standing on his own two feet as he calls it, and now we don't know for sure when Colin will be standing on his own two feet.

The effect on Colin's mother is that he is now in her mind almost the whole time; when he is at home she is focussed on him, and even if he is not in the room she is listening to the footsteps in the house in case he goes to the kitchen and then leaves it with something on the stove, because he forgets what he has just done. When he is out they worry constantly:

> You're on tenterhooks all the time wondering if he's on his way home, if he's safe. Colin can't understand that worry, he sees it as being overprotective...I mean I think he realizes that he's had this sort of accident, but he doesn't think it's worth worrying about. It's like somewhere it's closed down in his mind that it's happened and that's it. I don't know whether it's his way of coping with it.

Mr and Mrs White talk about Colin constantly 'he comes into nearly every conversation...we've always loved him and cared about him and we've always been there for him, but I suppose really this has really brought us closer together. Well, it either does that or it does the opposite doesn't it?'

Although sometimes she feels that she would like to break down, Mrs White feels that she is unable to let go:

> I get to a pitch and I think, oh I'd love a good howl and I just can't do it anymore because it seems, when you think 'oh, I'd love a good cry', you know, when you're sort of tensed up and that, everything else seems so mundane that it's not worth crying about anyway. So I just think, oh no, I

> won't waste my time and I just get on. I think sometimes I'm too tired to cry.

She is hoping that things will get better, gradually, and that she will not be faced with any more crises. But what emerges from this case history is that there is no point at which the family can sit back and feel that life is really back to normal. It is now three years since the accident, and these parents still feel they have no idea what is going to happen next, and the household is still very much affected by Colin's mood swings:

> If Colin is all right, we're all right, but if Colin is a bit uptight, we get quite tensed up, because you don't know what he might do and you don't know what mood he might be in; I mean it just goes by what ever mood he's in, that's what you go by...if you want to be truthful, emotionally, at the moment, he rules the household - and it's going to be ongoing, isn't it?

Violent emotions: 'Its like there's two people inside of me'

The Green family have a number of problems, different in many ways from those of the Whites, but similar to the extent that they also feel that at any stage that they think things are improving, something happens to turn their lives upside down again.

A year after his head injury Sam felt that, in many ways, he was progressing well; he was going to the local general hospital for rehabilitation one day a week, and had also returned part-time to the firm where he had been on a Youth Training Scheme course before his accident. At home, though, there were quite serious stresses and strains: his relationships with his brothers and sisters were now not very good, and his relationship with his father had changed, as Mrs Green explained:

> [His father] will sort of look on the black side of things...and I think after an accident like this Sam needs somebody to say, 'it's all right,' you know, 'things will get better,' and unfortunately he tends to do the reverse, he says 'you're going to end up with nothing' and that is not what he needs to hear. He has ended up with nothing as it is, and he certainly doesn't need that.

Sam himself feels that his father is very negative towards him, and that he has little understanding, especially compared with his mother:

> He just keeps telling me I'm bad, you know, I'm the sort of dirt beneath his shoe. It's not I don't like him, it's sort of the way he reacts and you

think, why the hell did you say that, you know. He's always putting me down. But [my mother] is about the most understanding person I know. Everything you find wrong with yourself she'll either put you right or she'll put you in the direction to get yourself right, so she'll help you get back to recovery.

Sam's father knows what Sam feels, but he says the things he does because he thinks it is for Sam's own good. He also wants to show Sam affection, but is afraid to be demonstrative:

> I think he thinks that anything I say is going to be against him, or something that he shouldn't do, or to try and get him away from something. I try and encourage him as much as I can - occasionally I'll put my arm round him and that sort of thing but you can see that he's uneasy when I do it, and I would rather not be like that than him sort of saying 'for Christ's sake', you know.

The most worrying thing that these parents were facing was Sam's new obsession with violence, and they were trying to discourage his passion for guns and knives. He watched violent videos, and played for hours with tiny model figures, many of them in the form of deformed monsters, which he painted with wounds and bullet holes and a great deal of blood and mangled flesh. Sam talked a great deal about violence and destruction. He obviously had a great deal of anger, which emerged in various ways, and was explicitly expressed in the reiterated questions: 'Why *me*? Why did it have to happen to *me*?' They were all worried, including Sam, that he might do something really violent, and if he did, as his father said: 'then he will be wearing that tag for the rest of his life'.

So far Sam had only been verbally aggressive, but his parents believed that he was probably capable of physical violence now. He would describe in graphic detail all the horrific injuries that he would like to inflict on people. This tended to upset his mother, and when she talked about the possibility that he might attack someone, she burst into tears.

Apart from these acknowledged problems, and changes in personality, Sam and his parents were quite optimistic at this stage, at least in terms of Sam's progress at work, and growing independence. Quite suddenly all this changed. Sam had his first epileptic fit since immediately after his accident, and although in some families the likelihood of a fit had been stressed, sometimes with the result that parents lived in daily dread of it happening, Sam's family say that although he had been prescribed an anticonvulsant drug for some months, no one at the hospital ever mentioned the possibility of fits to them.

This epileptic fit changed the whole situation; Sam's progress in the outside world suffered a severe setback and, at home, confidence and morale were low. His mother, no longer optimistic about the future, felt that Sam was trapped at home, and in the present:

> It's so unfair. It's almost like having a prison sentence, but not being imprisoned, if you know what I mean, which I sometimes think is worse - and for something which you haven't done. The basic accident itself...wondering whether he was going to wake up, that was bad enough but you can cope with that, but the fear of the unknown - you think you're going along fine and then something comes up and you think oh my God, back to square one, and it's that constant sort of stop and start that really plays havoc with you...particularly now - not at first, I was strong enough to cope - but it's really wearing me down now, and the longer it goes on the worse it gets [She starts to cry].

Sam also lost confidence, and was scared of having another fit, as his mother said:

> He had started back at college...and the more he went in the more excited he got about it, you know, he thought this is great, I can catch up with the bits that I've missed and I'll be able to start my second year in September, and he was really looking forward to that, but obviously he now feels that, well, you know, is that so certain? He said last night, 'I'm so frightened, what if I'm working with a saw and I have a fit and I lose my arm?' he said, 'I don't want to lose my arm.' So you see he obviously is frightened.

Although they tried hard to get hold of the hospital psychologist their efforts failed. Sam's mother became very depressed, but she was unsure how well her husband was coping because, she said, 'I've never really seen him sort of *unload*'. However, it was quite clear from Mr Green himself that he felt that the effects of the accident on the family, and on his relationship with his wife, were profound:

> After fourteen or fifteen years of marriage, we were getting very close and that sort of thing, and I was really enjoying marriage perhaps more than I had when we first started, and then, because of Sam needing you [to wife], like, the baby aspect...I'm not jealous that he'll go and see her rather than me, but perhaps that he's taking more of her time than he should do and perhaps, I hate to say it, but when we first got married we were that far apart [holding arms far apart] and then after fifteen years we were gradually, every year, getting closer like that [holding hands close together], and suddenly...its starting to go this way again [spreading

> hands out again]...that's the way that I look at it, but having said that, I know that he needs a lot of love, he needs to know that he's loved.

Mr Green cared about his son, but he wanted a future without him always around:

> The future is one of my very big concerns...there's no way in which I want Sam to be dependent on us, because we want to start enjoying ourselves now, we've had the children, we love the children dearly, we love Sam dearly, but we want a little time on our own. I think we would push - sorry, guide - him towards having his own place.

Both parents felt that Sam himself was worried about the future. His mother expressed it in terms of his awareness of what he could and could not do now. He saw his inabilities but 'doesn't want to admit to them'. This held him up at college because he was reluctant to ask for help, he said: 'I did it before, why can't I do it now?'. He tries hard to express himself but often finds it frustrating:

> I can't always bring out what I'm trying to say, I mean like now, I can see it up in my head but I can't get to it, I can't get what I want to say out and I can't get the feeling out.

His father pinpointed the uneasy limbo in which Sam, and many other young head injured people, find themselves: 'the fact that he is not able, but he's not *dis*abled, type of thing, he's in the middle, and he doesn't know what camp to go in. He wants to go into the able-bodied camp, but he can't because of epileptic fits'.

At this stage Mrs Green was very worried both by what Sam might do, and what might happen to him. She looked pale, even ill. Her husband said:

> She's very tired, yes, that is a really big concern for me, that it is taking a toll...I see it a darn sight more than other people do, and that might be tied in with this thing, you know that Sam is needing more of her attention and I'm not liking that, you know, psychologically.

Soon after this, Sam was asked to leave the college where he worked, because his behaviour was thought to be threatening to other students. He was then accepted on another course, at a different college, but this also came to an abrupt end when he was told that he was 'not up to scratch'.

Sam now felt even more anxious about the future, his chosen career seemed to be closed to him and he admitted he was scared, although he said that most of the time 'it just comes out as anger'. In fact his aggression continued to be a major problem, and Sam still felt that he might lose control if he was provoked:

I'm afraid I might do something violent; the two moves I would use, if it was a man I would knee him between the legs and then punch him in the solar plexus. That would do him for breathing for about five seconds. And he would be crippled and curled up on the floor in a lot of pain and then I'd just run away.

The anguish that Sam was suffering was very apparent, and in spite of his feeling that he could not express himself very well he in fact described his emotional state very graphically. At one point, when he was describing yet more ways of killing or crippling people, he suddenly stopped himself, and then said:

Just thinking about it, I think 'God, no, what are you thinking of?' It's like there's two people inside of me, once I've got past a certain point I just go, it's like a potion boiling over and suddenly this demon pops out...the anger that I feel inside me makes me want to go out and break somebody's neck. But [then] I just want to sit down, I want to be calm, I want to find out what's wrong with me...I can control the anger but in other ways it's sort of fighting me to get out.

Although he had been threatening at work, he had not yet been physically violent, but none of them, including Sam himself, knew whether this was because he had just not reached the point where he could no longer control it, as his mother said:

I think that's probably his fear and our fear, that is, how far can he take being pushed before he will blow his cool?

He and his parents were afraid that he might hurt one of his younger sisters and brothers, because his relationship with them had deteriorated rapidly. Everyone moved very carefully around him, scared to cross him in case he lost his temper.

His self-awareness was, in certain ways, very acute, and had a certain poignancy. Picking out one of the tiny mangled model figures, he held it up and said:

This is what I think of myself at the moment, I've got a chain saw strapped to one arm, a [laser?] gun strapped to the other and I've built all [this] incredible strong armour that takes a lot of shooting to get to it...that's what I think I am at the moment.

The family feel that the situation is endless. Sam's progress seems to have levelled off, his violent emotions are unabated, and their constant attempts over many months to get professional help have been unsuccessful. Objectively, what is happening in this family might have been expected - as the actual accident recedes in time other members of the family expect to return to a normal way of life. But Sam's life is far from normal, and his behaviour and emotions, which people made allowances for at first, are now hard to tolerate. His siblings are no longer prepared to put up with him; his father expects him to behave like a mature adult. Similarly, although the 'levelling off' process is inevitable, even Sam's mother feels let down in some way, because no one prepared them for this long, apparently endless, period of limbo.

Sam's future is very unclear. He is bitter about this because, from his point of view, the accident has totally changed his life. His main bitterness is still towards the man who knocked him down:

> Nobody else has really messed up my life or can mess up my life as badly as he has. I really do feel pretty hateful to the man - *everything*'s gone now, the whole thing, you know, it's just really taken everything away from me. I keep saying I'll get better but that takes time. If he gets away with it and gets out of court with me getting nothing, I'll probably spend the rest of my life in gaol after what I've finished doing with him.

Sam's current position is not an easy one for a nineteen year old. He has been thrown off two training courses, he is continually wracked by powerful and frightening emotions, and he feels that he is the 'odd one out' among people of his own age. The family as a whole is still dominated by the threat of violence.

One glaring fact that is apparent from this account is that Sam and his family are living under enormous strain, and no help appears to be forthcoming, in spite of repeated attempts to alert the professionals. The other members of the family feel they are always having to 'tread on eggshells' in their attempts not to upset Sam. They live with the constant insecurity of not knowing what will happen next, not only in terms of what Sam might do, but also, since his fit, they feel that nothing is certain any more. Relationships are strained between Sam and his sisters and brothers; his father finds it difficult to relate to him in a positive fashion, and resents the amount of attention he gets from his mother, and the effect that this is having on their marital relationship. Worst of all, perhaps, is the anxiety that Sam might commit some violent act, and that at any moment they might all be plunged into an even greater nightmare.

Father and son: 'You never ever give me a chance'

The chief problem in the Wiles family is the relationship that has developed between Jim Wiles and his father. Jim is eighteen, and was still living at home when he was head-injured. As in the case histories above, Jim resents the restrictions imposed on him by his parents, and his position is exacerbated by the hostility of his father. His parents say he has changed a great deal since his accident. Jim disagrees, though he does admit that he has sharp mood swings and that his memory is not very good, and that sometimes he feels quite aggressive.

Like Glenn and Colin, Jim feels that he should be independent of his parents, at least as far as the evenings are concerned. His parents say that when he stays out late at night, and gets tired, and whether he drinks alcohol or not, his movements become uncoordinated and his speech grows very slurred. His father, in fact, calls him a 'nuisance drunk' when he is in this condition, even if he knows he has not been drinking. Jim thinks that he is old enough to make his own decisions about what he does in the evening, especially now he is eighteen. But his father disagrees: 'Nobody, on your eighteenth birthday, sticks a key in your back and turns you into something different.' In fact his father disagrees with almost everything that Jim says. They argue and argue, with Mr Wiles trying to tie his son up in logical knots, and scoring points off him. Jim says his father will not let him say what he is trying to say, and 'puts him on the spot':

> You know that when I'm put on the spot, I get all things muddled up and I just say 'oh that's it' and just curl back up in my shell and you take advantage of that...I get embarrassed and then just curl into a ball and say 'no, it's all right'.

After one of these prolonged wrangles, Mr Wiles - in front of Jim and in fact directed at him - explodes violently:

> I'm beginning to bloody wonder whether it was ever worth while, the effort that I put into him...if he went backwards I could turn around to him and say, 'you put yourself there, you're an utter waste of time'. What annoys me is that he'll kid people that he's all right but it's all for his own end, and then suddenly he'll go straight to pieces...and then he'll say, 'well I have had a head injury'. But if I stood back and let him go his own way I would feel that I'd failed as his father, but this is where you're so self centred that the only thing that matters is you, and since the accident this is all that you get out of him, when it suits him: 'I've had an accident you know'.

Jim says to his father 'You never ever give me a chance'. He tries to put his point of view, when he can get a word in edgeways:

> I think that because of my head injury they [his parents] have lost confidence in me, they don't think I can do what I used to do, but I'm

near enough how I used to be...although I'm not 100 per cent how I used to be but it's near enough, it's getting better all the time.

Jim's father seldom seems able to empathise with his son. Most of the time he criticizes him as though he is still the same as he was before the accident, although he knows full well that he is not. He does acknowledge that Jim feels 'inferior'. This seems to upset him even more, because it is so vitally important to him, as his father, that he should not be inferior. He makes Jim feel even worse by shouting at him and showing him up in public, pointing out his faults and trying to confuse him, and then he seems to reach a point of exasperation and says impatiently: 'You're about as thick as a bloody dictionary'. There are moments, however, when Mr Wiles seems to relax his guard, and shows that he does understand that Jim has problems of his own:

> I have never known him spend so much time looking in the mirror...and I'll say to him 'what are you looking for Jim?' and I honestly think that he feels a bit inferior and he's looking for inferiority in himself...when he gets uncoordinated he'll go up to his room, he tries to shut it out; like with the mirrors, the way that he's feeling he's expecting to see it in his face. I've gone up to his room and he's been looking in the mirror and I say 'what do you see now?' and he'll say 'oh, something gorgeous!' you know, he passes it off as a joke.

The situation causes some tension between the parents, because his father feels that Jim has now become 'devious', and manipulates his mother: 'He does his best to exclude me', he said, 'If he wants hard advice he'll come to me, if he wants his own way he'll go to his mother'.

This sort of situation is found in many families, in normal circumstances, but may be exacerbated in families such as the Wiles, because of the mixture of conflicting emotions that each parent has towards their head injured child. Jim's mother, for example, is caught between husband and son, feeling sorry for Jim because he is still 'recovering' (though without really knowing what that means), nervous of what effect trying to restrict him will have on how he feels and behaves, and yet wanting him to be more cooperative. She is certainly less hard on Jim than his father is, and she defends him some of the time, but also tries to get Jim to see his father's point of view. At the same time she manages to slip her own criticisms and complaints about Jim into the father-son wrangles, to some extent under the umbrella of her husband's much harsher criticisms, so that hers seem relatively mild. When Jim goes on about being allowed out late at night, and after a long argument between Jim and his father, she says:

> Are we supposed to wait until you collapse? We've been told that when it's something to do with the brain that's something that could go wrong at any time...I mean we don't know, when he's out, whether anything's happened, you know, it's a total worry.

Like many other parents, having been told that something could 'go wrong' she is scared to let her son out of her sight for too long, although without knowing what it actually means. The only fear that is identifiable is of an epileptic fit, but for Mrs Wiles, as for many of the parents, an undefined miasma of anxiety has been conjured up by the imprecise warnings given at various times by professionals.

One of the problems that Jim recognizes is that he now has a 'short fuse', and is quickly angered. To begin with this was nothing more than a vague feeling of aggression, but something happened with one of his friends that frightened him:

> We were just having a muck around fight, and that, and just something twigged and I turned round and just sort of pinned him down and started strangling him, and I thought, you know, Jim, calm down. I just snapped, just like that, I was so wound up.

Jim's father had wanted him to have some psychological help from the beginning, but it was not until much later that a counsellor was provided. The hostility at home had been noted (in his medical records) before Jim originally came home, but it appears that the situation was then forgotten. This case history highlights an important aspect of life at home after a head injury. The young person who has had a head injury returns from hospital with many problems of his or her own. These often appear to be exacerbated by the reactions to them of other members of the family. The circumstances are new to everybody: the young person concerned, his or her father, mother, sisters and brothers. All the members of the household may need help to readjust and renegotiate their relationship with the head injured person, and also with each other.

Mother and daughter: 'She doesn't want me anywhere near her'

In some families there is an expectation that when their head-injured child returns from hospital he or she will fit into some kind of sick role, happy to be tended by loving parents. In reality this seldom, if ever, happens. Paula Gates was in a coma for two months after a road accident. Her parents brought her home as soon as they could, but were quite unprepared for what happened then. In the hospital, when they were all fighting for her to 'come back' her mother said 'it's rather like the war in a funny sort of way...you've got to fight, and you've got to keep each others' spirits up - and then suddenly you're left on your own, you're left to cope with it'. She says she used to think that if you loved someone absolutely it could 'conquer everything', but she soon came to realize that Paula did not want her to express her love:

> She said 'mummy' first [in the hospital] and I thought, oh right, we're home and dry. How *stupid* can you be. We weren't a bit home and dry, that was the start of it. I hadn't thought of the problems that we've been facing...anger all the time, anger about everything, whatever I say, and she doesn't want me anywhere near her, I can't kiss her or cuddle her, or show any love...she had broken away from us and she doesn't want to come back and be a child again, so she's fighting against it and I feel that's part of the anger against me. Also the fact that she can't do all the things she used to.

Thus instead of a daughter whom she could nurture and fuss over, Mrs Gates found herself with a highly difficult and unhappy person. She had thought that she would probably be a sort of invalid, and in a wheelchair. Asked if that would have been easier to cope with, Mrs Gates replied without hesitation: 'Yes, it would have been, isn't that a dreadful thing to say...yes, it would have been'.

Paula's anger was mainly focussed on her mother, though her constant anger, irritability and swearing affected everyone in the family. After a bit her mother began to prefer not to be left alone with her, 'at times I'm a little bit frightened of her'. Because Paula was so critical of her she found she was beginning to stammer, and when they were out in the car she found that her driving was affected. She went to her GP who prescribed antidepressants but, at that stage, no counselling or other help was offered. At one point, when Paula went back into hospital for an operation, her mother admitted to being relieved that she was not at home:

> While she's been in hospital it's been quite nice actually; in a dreadful guilty sort of way I do have to admit that. It's horrible to have to admit it isn't it? I said to her as I went, yesterday evening: 'looking forward to having you back, darling.' And I thought, you liar. Isn't that awful of me, I felt a hypocrite.

Paula's father also felt the strain, and he too was prescribed antidepressants. Mrs Gates said that he tended to say all the wrong things to Paula, because he was so nervous, and that since the accident he had 'sort of crumbled'. According to Paula, however, her father was better than before because, for the first time, he was 'being honest, not saying everything is marvellous'.

Much of the time, because they felt they could not react against Paula, her parents took it out on each other, snapping at each other, as Mrs Gates put it, 'like a couple of Jack Russells at each other's ankles'. Mr Gates said that his wife was the strong one, and that when he had contemplated suicide (for a number of reasons, including the situation with Paula) it was she who managed to drag him up out of what he called 'this beaten misery'. Mrs Gates herself did not feel particularly strong much of the time, and had felt at times as though she was quite out of control:

> I'm not strong, I can only be strong for little bits at a time and then all of a sudden I go quite mad and I can't take any more and I have about three or four days where I'm completely off the rails basically...I can't cope, and then I'm back on the rails again, and this is how my life seems to be going, it's a dreadful admission, but I mean I just can't keep going on the rails, day in and day out.

For almost a year after the accident she tried to cope on her own, and tried not to let people know how near to collapse she was:

> I was getting really down, in fact the whole family was falling apart at the seams really then a friend...took me to one side and said, 'how are you coping?' And I suddenly thought, I'm sick of saying 'oh fine' and laughing, and I said, 'I'm not, I'm not coping, the whole thing's falling apart.'

Paula herself was aware that she was behaving in a difficult way, but resented the way her parents were treating her:

> Mum and Dad are treating me as if I'm about ten again. They're driving me mad, they're treating me as though I'm some sort of invalid. I'm supposed to be normal again now. I love it when she goes out and leaves me on my own, it's freedom...I think she finds it hard to leave me alone, let go, but I need a bit of space sometimes to breathe.

During this period Paula made at least one suicide attempt. She described one:

> I walked in front of a car and the bloody thing stopped, could you believe it. Just my luck, I can't even kill myself and get it right...I got pissed and then thought I'll walk in front of a car, why not? I wanted to end it all.

Although this was apparently done on the spur of the moment, Paula's mother said that she had often said she would rather be dead, and she believes that she did mean it at times. Before the accident Paula had been a lively, successful young woman. Now she was unable to do the things had come so easily before, and she also felt that she had been made physically ugly by her injuries, although these injuries are not in fact apparent to observers.

About fifteen months after the accident things settled down to some extent. Mrs Gates said 'She's not quite the old Paula, but almost'. There was less friction in the house, although Paula was still having severe mood swings, and her parents said that everything still revolved around her - she was in control, as her father said, 'You can't help censoring what you say'. Her mother still found herself fussing round Paula: 'I've got into this awful rut where I can't stop the anxiety, the non-stop anxiety.' Paula started driving again, and began making plans to leave home, but life had changed, and Mrs Gates felt that nothing would ever be the same as it had been before:

> It'll never be quite the same again, never. Relationships will never be the same again, there's a certain naivete has died. We'd been always skating on the surface, because we never actually got involved with anything too dreadful...we never really had to come face to face with actual life.

Not only had the course of their lives been changed, but Paula herself, in her mother's view, was no longer the same person that she had been before:

> There are sort of differences that you can't put a finger on really...she tends not to react as you think she's going to; it's as if there is a different person in there really. Whether or not the old person will ever come back, I don't know, I think probably not. So we've just got to like the new person. But she isn't the same.

Just under two years after the accident Paula went travelling abroad. Although her mother was miserable when she first went, she found that she was gradually beginning to feel better: 'more like me'. Left to themselves, she and her husband now get on 'like a house on fire'. She still has symptoms of anxiety, and continues to take antidepressants, but life has returned, to a great extent, to the calmer days of before the accident. The worry about Paula is still there in the background, but is decidedly less acute in her absence:

> To be perfectly honest one half of me would love to see her again and give her a cuddle and the other half says no, it's so much simpler without her...I can now please myself, I can live my life really...all the things I want to do, I'm now beginning to do. When she was here, we couldn't enjoy ourselves, if she went out in the car I was always worried until she came back, and then she'd be cross and bad tempered and then I'd think

> 'oh God, why doesn't she go out again?' and then I'd worry again. It was a sort of nightmare.

Mother and son: 'You can get on your own two feet'

In the Smith family, the divorced mother had become engaged since her son's accident, and this new relationship has tended to push the head injured son out of the household unit. His mother cared for him very devotedly for the first few months, taking a long period off work to be with him. He had begun to attend various courses at the local college, and spent some time at Headway. Some eighteen months later, however, his mother was spending much of the week away from home, and was hoping that Neville would soon be going away on a residential course:

> I think he should leave home, I'd say he's ready for the plunge. That might sound all very sort of cool, but I feel the time has come that he should stand on his feet...I think, probably, he feels he hasn't got much of a home life, I very rarely see him, I don't know what he does, he's very secretive, I don't question where have you been, what are you doing and that sort of thing. Maybe that to him might be, well, I'm not interested. I spend a lot of time where my partner is...so I do split my life and I have to admit it's like a form of escape.

Neville appeared to be able to look after himself, although his memory was still not very good. He was very solitary and withdrawn, and his moods tended to swing from high to low very quickly. His mother said that he was rude and obstinate, and said: 'I ignore him'. She felt that she got on less well with him than she had before, and frequently became impatient and frustrated with him. She was keen to start afresh: 'I've got a new life, a new beginning, and I don't want it to fail'. She felt that everything she did for Neville 'he would throw back in your face and just treat you like dirt'.

Many parents in the study felt that their help and support was often thrown back in their face, but persevered because they felt that this was part of the effects of the head injury, and thus not their children's fault - though it was often hard to bear. In Mrs Smith's case, however, her son's behaviour was taken almost as a justification for leaving him, and keeping her new life separate from him. She said that Neville was 'not the same person that he was' and 'doesn't understand where his loyalties lie within the family'. Neville, however, said that he would like to live with his mother when she finally moved in with her fiancé, but said 'I don't think she wants me to live with them. She said "you can get on your own two feet now and get out"'.

He did not appear to mind very much, he said he was not close to his mother any more anyway. Altogether, he said, he felt different. He looked for support outside the home - he liked going to the day centre because: 'they're more concerned, more helpful than my mum is'.

A few months later Neville went on a residential course some distance from home. The family house was sold, his mother remarried and moved into a flat with her new husband. Although Neville came for some weekends she was trying to ensure that he would not come back and live with them. She hoped that he would stay in the town where his college was, but failing that she would find an alternative place for him to go. She has not been to visit him, and she says it is for her, to some extent, 'out of sight, out of mind'.

There is another mother who has a similar attitude to Mrs Smith's. Again, a new relationship has taken over, and she is hoping to move to another part of the country to live with her boyfriend. Although these are the only two parents who have taken this action, they are not unique in their feelings. Many of the other parents in the study feel that it is time that they were allowed to get on with their own lives, but continue as they are because they feel they have no justification for changing the situation. Some have no choice; in one family, where the daughter is still unable to walk, and needs constant care, the parents feel that their life together, to do the things they wanted to do, will never happen, as the mother says: 'We get angry with the situation for the simple reason it took all these years to start having a life of our own, Lou and I, now it's gone again...that's why I feel bitter'.

What is remarkable is not that two single mothers have decided to live their own lives (in both cases more than a year after the accident), but that so many families are prepared to continue to focus very largely on their head injured son or daughter for so long, and with very little support or advice from anyone else. Part of this willingness to continue is based on a thankfulness that their son or daughter is still alive. One woman's son, some two years after his accident, is still having problems which disrupt the whole household - drinking too much, being physically aggressive (to her and to his brothers), having violent mood swings, and so on. But, as his mother graphically describes, the only important thing is that he is alive:

> He nearly died, and the feeling inside, in here, is that he was nearly taken away from me. When I'm driving sometimes, and I pat him on the knee, 'You're doing it again, mother,' he says, 'I'm still here - I'm not going to disappear in a puff of smoke'. But all I can say is that you are touching somebody who is warm, it's the only way you can put it; touching him, he's *warm*, and I know that he could have been cold, you see, dead. I still

do it, but not as much as I used to [she begins to cry]. I dreaded feeling him, and that he'd be cold.

3 The family: sisters and brothers

The effects that a severe head injury has on one member of a family necessarily have a wide range of interconnected repercussions on the rest of the family. The sisters and brothers of the head injured sibling find that not only are their emotions affected by the initial experience of seeing their brother or sister in a coma in hospital, and then by his or her return to live within the household, but also by the emotions and behaviour of their parents, and of each other. In addition, for weeks and probably months, life in the household is in a state of continual upheaval. In fact, this disruption may continue, to a lesser, but significant extent - for years, and involves realignments and renegotiation of all the relationships within the family.

Some degree of change in relationships between the head injured member of the family and his or her brothers and sisters was apparent in all the families. Although the sibling relationships that existed before can only be gauged from reports after the event, it seems that in most cases the relationship has become less close. The changes that take place do not seem to be related to physical injuries; the friction that tends to develop between sisters and brothers appears to be more directly related to changes in personality, however subtle and hard to identify these may sometimes be. Each sibling relationship will also be inextricably bound up with all the other interrelationships between various members of the family, and each will be directly and indirectly affected by the return to the household of a young person who has suffered a severe head injury. How each sister or brother reacts will depend not only on the interaction between him or herself and the injured sibling, but also upon the emotions and behaviour of each parent, of other siblings, of the amount of support that is given from outside sources and so on. In addition to this web of relationships there are also specific factors that will affect siblings, such as the degree of guilt, based on fact or fiction, regarding the accident itself, the individual characteristics of the earlier relationship, the relative ages of the siblings and the severity of the effects of the injury.

'I don't like to see a family split'

In some families the young head injured person and his or her siblings find it difficult to resolve the hostility that arises between them. Before they realize what is happening they are caught up in an emotional tangle which may veer from mutual abusiveness to a refusal to have anything to do with each other. In the Morgan family, for example, there had been trouble between the sisters and brothers since Darren came home from hospital three months after his accident, although it had perhaps been brewing even before he came home. Darren turned against his siblings, and after a year of trouble, this became almost impossible for his mother to bear. Darren had been living away from home before the accident, but afterwards came home to live with his parents. His brother, Des, lives away from home, and he and Darren, and their respective girlfriends, became locked in battle, while their mother sat at home - losing weight, getting headaches and feeling totally drained - worrying about the fighting, and not knowing what she could do to bring her family together. 'I think it's basically because no one really understands what happens with head injuries' she said:

> Darren has this thing in his head that everyone is against him...he is the worst one deep down because he's got so much resentment and he won't be talked to.

Although she realized the cause of the friction, she was unable to persuade her other children to ignore Darren's hostile behaviour. They took it personally and reacted against him, in spite of the effect that this was having on their parents, especially their mother:

> I don't like to see a family split up when they've been so close. I mean it seems to hurt me; I can't live a normal life because it's there all the time. I go to bed and I think about it and I get up in the morning and it's still there, it's on my mind and it's like something crushing down on you, I can't explain the feeling, because although I might appear to be all right, it's there.

It was the relationship between the brothers, each supported by his girlfriend, that was the most difficult, with accusations and abuse flying in both directions. Darren's mother bottled up her anxiety; she tried not to talk to her husband about it because it tended to lead to arguments. She also felt that she could not really tackle Darren about it because she had no idea know what effect it would have on him, although at first she did try:

> He was rude, really aggressive, and I think I was probably down myself, at the time, and I couldn't cope with it properly, so several times we had rows...then I tried - because I was always worried he would have an epileptic fit. I still keep from saying things sometimes because I don't want him to have a fit. I mean there's always the chance, isn't there, if he gets too stressful; when he gets into one of his moods I can't explain the look on his face - and the real anger, that's another thing, things like that, if only we knew what we *could* say.

No one had explained anything to Darren's parents, or talked to them about the kinds of problems that could arise, and to make things worse, they lived in constant fear - as many parents did - that if they upset their son he might have a fit, or something equally worrying. Although they had seen a psychologist at the very beginning, in the hospital, since he had been home they had had no help or advice: 'we're left high and dry really'. His mother partly blamed herself for not seeking help:

> I feel I've done wrong; instead of keeping it in, if only I'd have done something about it, not let it go on and think, oh well probably it'll be all right by tomorrow, perhaps something will happen...you sort of feel to blame don't you? If I had gone to the doctor perhaps he could have put me in touch with someone.

Her husband did not agree; he felt that their children had got to sort it out between themselves:

> Yes, OK, we can talk to whoever we want to and, like, we're talking to you, but it doesn't solve no problems, does it? Yes, OK, we'll go to counsellors and we'll go to the high court, but it'll solve no problems - it's the children who have got to do the talking, not us.

Darren himself, although happy to be interviewed, was unwilling to say very much about his current relationships with his siblings, he said it was 'too personal'. All he would say is: 'I feel strongly what I think, but perhaps that's the head injury playing tricks, I don't know'. He says he does not care much about what other people are feeling 'as long as I'm all right'.

A few months later the situation had eased to some extent. Mrs Morgan had been to see her GP who had given her antidepressants, and arranged for her to see a counsellor. Her children had 'made it up', and although they still did not see each other, the fact that they *said* they had made it up was a real comfort to her.

However, two months after this it was clear that the situation had not really changed. Darren had married his girlfriend, and had not invited his brother to the wedding. But the fact that Darren no longer lived at home meant that his mother no longer had to face the problem on a daily basis. She had stopped taking antidepressants, and was certainly less depressed than she had been a few months earlier. She had managed to cope with the fact that her son had had a severe head injury, but the effect that this was having on her family was harder to bear:

> I could quite easily have committed suicide, that's the way I felt, because it seemed like my whole life had been shattered really. I know there is people worse off than me, but it didn't seem to help. I tried to see it that way, but this was my family and it was hurting.

For Darren's mother, being interviewed in this research project made her realize that something *could* be done to help her. Although the project itself was unable to provide what she really wanted, it made her feel that she was not alone in the world - which was how she had felt before:

> That was sort of like an opening to me when you came, just to talk to someone. I thought, oh this is really brilliant, I was so pleased, although you couldn't [help?], you can listen, which is a great help; but when you first came I thought, oh you was going to do so much for me and you was going to sort it all out for me and everything was going to be a bed of roses; and you did help because just talking, that really made a lot of difference...and then I had my counsellor, but it's not the same as being here, in your own home chatting to someone, though I mean she was very nice, I couldn't fault her at all.

Her distress seemed to go unnoticed by the professionals she came into contact with when she took Darren in to the hospital for his various appointments. It is true that she probably did not tell them what was happening, but it would only have taken one sympathetic word to have evoked a reaction that would have been hard to ignore:

> It would have helped, and also as a family, I think if someone had been there and just spoken to us all and explained what might happen - it's as if you were non-existent - if there had been someone there to *explain*. [The consultant] said he'd have memory problems and sort of like bad mood swings but there was nothing else, how to *cope* with that. If they could help people more, you know *talk* to them, it would save things like this [trouble at home] happening, because I wouldn't wish it on anybody.

The trouble between the sisters and brothers in this family might not have been totally avoidable, but would have been helped if all the members of the family had had more explained to them at a very early stage. Hostility between them and Darren's girlfriend's family, which began at the bedside when Darren first had his accident, was a contributing factor to the situation, and this, too, might have been defused if there had been a sympathetic intervention at the very beginning.

'People think I'm stupid'

In a situation where siblings have always been competitive and to some extent jealous of each other the effect of a head injury to one of them may lead to a temporary cease fire, but when life at home gets back to some sort of normality, the sibling rivalry may not only return, but be intensified.

In the Jones family the friction between Danny and his brother Keith had become very marked. Although Danny had recovered from his accident to a large degree, he still had weakness in one arm and leg, and had not yet been given back his driving licence (a very significant rite of passage for many of these young people). At one point Keith was also living at home, and relations between the two brothers were very bad. In fact Keith found himself in somewhat of a cleft stick. When Danny was well enough to want to go out to the pub Keith would take him there. What often happened on these outings was that Danny would feel that Keith was trying to limit his drinking, because he had been told that Danny should not drink too much, and, according to Danny 'he tells people I'm brain-damaged' to explain away any apparently odd behaviour. Both these things upset Danny, whereas Keith thought he ought to be grateful to Keith for looking after him, stopping him getting into fights, helping him in crowded bars, and so on. He said he made sure that Danny was all right, helped him to get through the crowds to the toilet, and so on. But according to Danny, Keith did this in such a way that it drew attention to him:

> People think I'm stupid. You were saying, 'get out of the way, my brother's disabled.' What did I say to you, Keith? 'can you walk in front of me to move people out of the way,' not advertise the fact that I'm disabled...you can explain to them, not 'he's a scared cripple'.

This made Keith angry:

> I asked people to move out of the way. See, he talks out of his arse. It's so annoying, sometimes I just don't want to bother with you at all...I don't *need* to help you at all. I mean it would be a whole lot less for me to do if I didn't have to worry about you or chase around town looking for you or whatever else.

Keith felt that all he got was abuse from Danny, in spite of his efforts to be 'brotherly', taking him out with his friends.

Although Danny resented Keith, he knew that he still needed him when he was out in a crowded place. He put on an act of bravado, but in fact he got very nervous, and Keith seemed to refuse to accept that his brother really was nervous. For example, on one occasion, when he had to find a telephone, Danny did not want to go round the pub asking where it was 'I just couldn't handle that', he said. Keith said he was being childish, 'you're turning into a baby, Dan', he said. Keith did not realize how difficult it was for Danny to walk across the room, through all the people, and ask the bartender a question. He taunted him, and kept insisting that Danny was not really nervous in the pub. Danny said furiously:

> That's what really pisses me off - Keith thinking he knows best about how I feel. When I'm in a crowded pub I do get nervous, you know, I can't help that, I *do* feel very uncomfortable and I can't handle it...I don't need people saying you're too weak to do that, you're too feeble to do that, you're too scared to do that. If I am a bit scared or nervous about it, that's me, isn't it, it's not for someone to say 'just do it mate, you're tough enough.' I don't need that at all.

When his brother was not there to hear, Danny said that Keith had always had an inferiority complex, and that that was why he reacted as he did. Danny said it was because he, Danny, had always been better at pulling the girls. Part of this Danny attributed to the fact that his hair was much longer than Keith's. When he had his accident his hair had been chopped right off when he was admitted to hospital:

> When I had my hair cut off he saw that as his head start, like his push, you know, in the right direction. Now my hair's grown back, it's getting the same again. He sees me coming back to my old self, he doesn't like it...if somebody cut my hair off again, I mean, people have sort of said it jokingly, I don't know what I'd do, probably kill 'em, but there's so many jealous people around, since my hair's grown back...I'm just paranoid of someone cutting it off again, when I'm asleep or something.

Dan's hair is symbolic of his identity and power, and as it grows he regains them both:

> If my hair hadn't been cut off I'd have been better ages ago, wouldn't I? That's what I was really cut up about my accident...things like my walking and my arm and stuff like that I knew was going to come back, and I know my hair's going to come back but it's going to take longer

isn't it? But that's what is really upsetting me, more than anything. I know it's only hair but it's part of my life. It's me, really.

Danny is not alone in equating his hair length with 'normality'. The importance of growing hair back to its previous length was brought up by some of the other young people who had woken up to find that their hair had been chopped off. In another family hair length was, as in Danny's case, a cause for sibling rivalry:

> He's fretful about his hair, that's all really, because it was very long, and he goes on and on about his brother's hair...'he's got really lovely hair and I want hair like that again,' he's very fretful about his hair, wanting to grow it again, but of course it would take him ages, he's not consoled by the thought that it will grow eventually.

'I might as well not have a brother'

In some families, hostility between siblings was caused less by rivalry than by a sibling's anger that the person with a head injury had brought such suffering to the family. This makes the family circumstances even more difficult. Even if there is some confusion about how the accident actually occurred, the person who suffered the accident, whatever the cause, would obviously not have intended or wanted to come through it with a head injury. Nevertheless, in the Webb family, for example, the overriding attitude of the non-injured brother, Ken, was that Cliff had 'messed up' all their lives. This attitude brought intense sadness to their mother:

> He won't forgive Cliff for what he's done, he said he hasn't just ruined his own life, he's ruined ours as well. He said 'you should have had a lot more sense'; in his eyes Cliff has just sort of thrown away all his opportunities, and other people's opportunities too, because like he said, we've worked hard to sort of give him the best. He said 'I might as well not have a brother.' [Mrs Webb starts to cry]

Mrs Webb feels that there is also an element of resentment. Ken has always sorted out his own problems, and 'he can't see why Cliff should have everybody running circles round him'. However, the main emotions seem to be anger, and sadness:

> It will be a continual grief for Ken...we were trying to explain to him that we were all feeling [the same], and saying 'we've all got to try' and he said, 'mum, I have lost my brother.'

This feeling was also expressed in other families: one sister said, when her brother was constantly hostile towards her: 'I don't care, he's not my brother any more'. Such statements carry a number of messages: my brother has changed; he is no longer the brother that I knew and cared about before, therefore he is not my responsibility. To some extent this may be a strategy to make the situation more bearable: if he is not my brother then I don't *have* to care about him. In Ken's case, it is also a disowning of someone who has behaved in what he feels is an unforgivable and 'unbrotherly' way: there are ways that brothers behave, and do not behave. It is perhaps reminiscent of the way that small children, when angry with their mother, say: 'you are not my mother, you are my wicked step-mother'. But as Cliff's mother says, there is also a note of anguish in what he says: 'I have lost my brother'.

'Its made the others grow up a lot'

In the families discussed above the young person with a head injury is walking and talking, and the hostilities, where they arise, can be acted out on both sides. But in families where the person is, in a sense, unable to enter into such a relationship, the reactions of brothers and sisters may be quite different. Stephie Bell is unable to walk, and as yet able to speak only a few words. She lives in the centre of a large and active family, consisting of her parents, a number of older sisters and brothers who either live there or are constantly in the house, grandparents, sisters-in-law and brothers-in-law, nieces and nephews, who all come and go throughout the day. Mrs Bell feels that the accident has changed her other children:

> Its made the others grow up a lot more and they're grateful for each other now. They appreciate life, I think, now, that's what it's done to them. I think, once something happens in the family it does make them a lot different.

Because of the severity of the results of the accident none of the siblings are openly hostile towards her, though some find it easier to relate to her than others do. The eldest sister, Rose, for example, has taken on a motherly role, putting Stephie first, even before her husband. By contrast, another sister 'can't cope with Stephie - she comes and sees her, but she won't do the things with her like Rose will'. Thus the two sisters have reacted in very different ways. One has become motherly and supportive, supplementing the mother's nursing role, but the other has cut herself off, not exposing herself to the strain of trying to deal with Stephie's needs, or the frustration of trying to work out what Stephie is trying to communicate.

Similarly one brother now spends time with Stephie, although before they were said to be 'always at loggerheads', whereas another one, who has always been very close to Stephie, refuses to do things for her, such as feeding her, because by doing so 'he feels he is treating her as a baby, and he doesn't like it'. It is this youngest son that their mother thinks has been the most neglected. He was sixteen when the accident happened, and from then on he was very much expected to behave like an adult. He himself said he felt that he had been neglected since Stephie's accident 'they're always pushing me away' he said, and it is clear that he is the one who has lost out the most in terms of day to day attention from his parents. At the same time he has found that his outside activities have been seriously curtailed: his mother insists on knowing where he is all the time, and tries to keep him at home as much of the time as possible.

Many of these parents, who have lived through the experience of one child suffering a severe head injury, become prey to anxiety about the safety of their other children in the outside world. Their ears are constantly reacting to the distant sounds of ambulance and police sirens - what was unthinkable has happened, and thus can happen again.

'I just felt I wasn't needed'

The reactions of parents when one of their young adult children suffers a severe head injury, and how they behave both to that child and to their other children, can have a devastating effect on the sisters and brothers of the one who has been head injured. The siblings have to contend not only with the hard task of coming to terms with what has happened to a brother or a sister, but also have to face a sometimes quite radical change in the behaviour and emotional focus of their parents. This situation is very apparent in the Taylor family.

When Geoff Taylor had his accident he had already been living away from home for some time, working in various jobs in different parts of the country. His sister, Jean, lived in a neighbouring village, not far from the parental home, with her husband and small children. Before the accident she said that she and Geoff were very close indeed, probably more so because there had been some sort of a rift between him and their parents, so he visited his sister often. After the accident, however, Jean found herself feeling very isolated, not only from Geoff, but also from her parents:

> I felt that I wasn't needed anymore...I went to the hospital, mum and dad didn't really explain to me immediately what had happened or the consequences of what had happened, so I just thought, as anyone would

think, head injury, bump on the head, he's lost his memory, you know, simple. So I went to the hospital and it wasn't until we sat down with the doctor and he explained everything that had happened, it really hit home, you know. And then for a while I was suspended, I didn't know what to think or do. I think for a while my own family suffered a bit, because I was torn between being there and here...for a while I went every day and then after a while I was afraid to go. I just felt spare. It was an odd feeling...I just hated seeing him like it and mum and dad seemed very close and I seemed outside.

She also, in those first days, had a row with her father. She realized it was partly because they all needed some release from the emotional tension, but it intensified her feeling of isolation. Geoff's accident appeared to have brought her parents closer, but she still feels herself to be on the outside, because they are now so focussed on Geoff:

> They've got Geoff at home now and sometimes I feel that that's all they need. While he was in hospital they didn't really come to see me, they went to the hospital, which I mean, you know, is obvious, but that's another reason I think I felt a bit - you know, just put to one side, put a bit on hold until things got better...I didn't feel close to them, I just felt a bit isolated for a while. It was very horrible. I just felt I wasn't needed; they spent every moment they had in the hospital, and I think I resented that in a way because they didn't come to see the children. The children got left out as well...I didn't blame them, I didn't hate them for it or anything, I just felt that they should really come and see the children.

There is, in many normal sibling relationships, an element of rivalry for the affection of parents, especially that of the mother (Firth, Hubert and Forge 1970: 426). The sudden, and almost total, focus of attention on a child, of whatever age, who suffers a severe head injury, can stir up this old rivalry, and unless parents are very careful, can unintentionally cause the well siblings to feel rejected and unloved.

In Jean's case there was also her own reluctance to take any of the burden from her parents in the early stages of recovery. She found it very hard to see Geoff when he was still in a coma, and when he started thrashing about as he came round she was afraid:

> I hated visiting him, I went, but I hated it...I was frightened of him. When he [changed hospitals] he was still unconscious but he used to shout, you know, he'd get really violent and I really hated it. I was frightened, not of him, I was just frightened that he might be like that when I got there. I used to wake up in the night screaming, it was awful, I used to have nightmares. We were told then it was very unlikely that he would live,

> and that he could be a cabbage for the rest of his life, the future looked really glum. That was when it really struck me, so, you know, it was very difficult to cope with. Luckily I had lots of friends around me, they were very supportive, the lady I work with, she used to sit there and listen to me going on and on.

One of the problems for the sisters and brothers in these circumstances is that the person they would normally turn to for support and strength is their mother, but because of the nature of the situation she is the one person that cannot be turned to. In Jean's case, she was lucky to have an extremely supportive husband and an employer who would listen.

Jean's parents said that they thought that some of her immediate reaction was because she felt she was to blame. All Jean herself said about this was 'if only' she had been with him that evening, she would have driven him home, and it would not have happened. Mrs Taylor said:

> We had a dreadful time with her didn't we? It was absolutely dreadful when it first happened. She for some reason blamed herself, as if it was her fault, and I don't know why she ever got that impression. She actually literally one night went completely over the top. She hit herself, she punched the walls she did everything, she was trying to hurt herself...she literally tried to really hurt herself. We had to really restrain her.

In spite of all this, there were obviously many times, in the days that followed the accident, that Jean and her parents sat together and talked. When Geoff was still in a coma, all of them thought at one point that it would be better if he died. Jean felt that, at the time, it would have been easier to cope with his death, than with the harrowing and long drawn out ordeal that survival involved - an emotion also expressed in other families - although she felt that it would have been 'an easy way out':

> When he was in hospital, especially when he was in the coma on the life support machine thing, then I did because it was the unknown. We didn't know to what extent he had brain damage, they basically said that he was going to be a cabbage for the rest of his life, so here we were sat there thinking well what on earth happens in the future? There were quite a few times when mum and dad and me, all of us, said it might have been better if he hadn't survived. But now we're glad he did. It's just the unknown I think. But I think we could have coped with that *better*, at the time. We could have grieved and it would have been gone, but because it went on and on and on for such a long time - the grief was so deep, it just went on and on.

Geoff, contrary to the early prognosis, recovered extremely well. To Jean, though, he still seems very different from before:

> To me he's still awful because he's nothing like he was before, but to someone who didn't know him before the accident, they probably wouldn't know a lot of difference - but he is totally different. Before he was wild, really, although I loved him...but now he's completely the opposite. I mean he was always nice but he had this wild streak, he didn't seem to care about anyone's feelings but now he's lovely.

Geoff himself feels he has changed, and that he is now quite unlike all the friends that he used to have:

> I feel different, I feel that I'm not the same as everybody else, sort of totally different. I used to be, as I remember, out drinking, heavily drinking, smoking, and acting - jokes and everything, I'm not like that any more. It's strange but it's different.

Jean's feelings for Geoff have also changed. To some extent she treats him with more caution:

> I'm not *frightened* of him but I'm careful about what I say to him, whereas before we would tease one another and joke...I think I care more about him now. Before he was a friend, he was my brother, but now, yes I do feel different, I care more, I worry about his feelings more. I shouldn't really, I suppose, he's just a normal person, but that's how I feel.

One of the new emotions she feels for him is compassion, especially when he was nervous and unsure of himself in public, and he seemed to feel that he had to make excuses for himself:

> He tells people he is head injured. He uses the expression head injured. He'll tell everyone...and I used to feel sorry for him that he'd have to make excuses for himself; I used to say, 'you don't have to say that, you're no different.'

Does she still grieve for him?

> I don't grieve for what he was before no. He's going to be what he's going to be and there's nothing we can do to change that. We can just help him to get better but we can't make him be what he was like before.

Every time she sees him now (some two years after the accident), which is about every two or so weeks, she sees a great improvement in him. Her relationship with her parents is improving, and she hopes that it will get back to 'normal' when Geoff becomes more independent, although she believes that it will be very hard for her parents to let him go, and start living a more normal existence.

Although she is not exactly jealous of Geoff, she is, in a sense, jealous of the whole situation. It may have been made worse, in part, by the fact that before the accident she saw much more of her brother than her parents did. As their mother said:

> I didn't even think about him - he knew where we were and he would find us if he needed us...we wouldn't see him for months, but we never bothered, never worried about him, he had his own life.

Now Geoff and his parents are very much a self-sufficient unit, and Jean is not being allowed to take any real responsibility for Geoff. They are, in some ways, treating him as though he is their only child, and by doing so they are not only making Jean feel excluded, but also to some extent preventing Geoff and Jean from returning to being a normal brother and sister. Jean and her husband want to help Geoff become more independent, they would have him to stay with them but her parents will not let him go. Jean says that if you ask him something they even answer for him, though he is quite capable of answering for himself.

Jean is sad for her parents because she knows that they have no close kin that they can talk to, and she says sadly: 'They've got me, if only they'd use me a bit more often'. Part of the trouble is probably because of her reactions in the early days. Her mother says that they had not been able to leave Jean with her brother: 'she would never stay with him on her own'. Now Jean is happy to stay with him, as her parents know, and would like him to come and spend some time with her and her family. She is worrying less about the future, but she spoke of a time, when Geoff was still in hospital, when she had become very anxious about what her responsibilities might be in the years to come:

> I felt very selfish, but I used to think, what would happen in the future if...he was conscious but not able to do things? I mean everyone expects to look after older relatives in later life but nobody expects to look after their brother for the rest of their life. And possibly for him to outlive us, and then our children to have to cope with him when he's really, you know, probably at one of his worst stages...It does cross my mind now and again that perhaps one day he will have to come and live with us...I'm being selfish again, but I think it'll be very difficult because you do need your own space, I mean, I think he needs his own space really.

She knows her parents will have him for a long time yet, if it is necessary, though the probability of Geoff living with some degree of independence becomes greater as the months pass. She realizes that her parents no longer have *their* own space, and she felt guilty that the possibility of having to look after her brother in later years should provoke so much anxiety in her. Like many other sisters and brothers in the same circumstances, she is having to confront, for the first time, the problem of identifying the limits and parameters of sibling responsibilities and rights.

'I feel guilty that I ignore her sometimes'

Cassie and Adam Lange were both still at school when Cassie suffered a severe head injury, and their relationship had been very close, though competitive as well. Cassie was very impressed when she heard that Adam had sat beside her in hospital, reading to her, and when she came home she said he was 'absolutely brilliant', and not too jealous that she was getting all the attention. In fact Adam found it difficult to know how to treat her:

> I do worry about her. I feel guilty that I ignore her sometimes...I suppose I don't really pay her enough attention, and I shouldn't really snap back at her so much, as well, because I know it's probably the accident that makes her snap but it's hard...because we've always got on very well, but it's always been quite a sort of competitive, aggressive relationship and it's hard to change something like that...it's hard to stop competing and sort of try and help her - but without letting her know I'm helping her, which makes it a false relationship anyway.

Their father thinks that it would have been easier for Adam if Cassie was in a wheelchair 'if there were something obvious to see physically he would find it a lot easier'. Adam also says:

> I suppose in some ways it would have been easier in the short term because then at least you could treat them like another person. It would be someone who would be dependent...not someone who you're trying to help who is pulling away at the same time, which I think is a lot of the problem.

The relationship between Cassie and Adam epitomises the dilemma in which many sisters and brothers find themselves. Because their head injured sibling has changed, the nature of the relationship also has to change. Adam, for example, feels that he has to treat Cassie differently, but wants it to remain an honest relationship, not one in which he is acting a part. On the other hand he does not feel that he should react to her bad temper as he would have in the past. Thus he tends to avoid the situation as much as he can.

Other siblings feel this reluctance to create a different relationship, and may grieve for the sister or brother that they used to have. One mother describes one of her son's reactions to his head-injured brother:

> He was like frightened of him. He couldn't sit still with him, he would sit still for five minutes and talk to him and then he would get up and wander away. He couldn't sort of get back into that good old relationship, you know, of two brothers, like they used to be - he couldn't cope with seeing him disabled, seeing him sort of struggling to walk.

In another family a younger brother took turns with his parents at the bedside of his brother, Joe, in hospital, and remained calm and patient for some months after Joe came home. Then, as his brother recovered, he began to react to the months of strain:

> He stayed all right for about four months, almost until Joe was okayish and then it felt like it was all right for him to blow a gasket, which he proceeded to do - he was awful...he was on drugs, he was uncontrollable, he wouldn't contribute, he was never in, he would never tell us where he was, I mean, he was rebelling totally, but the minute Joe went away he reverted to being fairly human really...no doubt he was going through a stage as well, but the extreme reactions were from sitting in that intensive care ward for two months at seventeen years old, watching his brother.

From these case histories it can be seen that there are many different reactions and problems that follow the severe head injury of a sister or brother, and the examples described are by no means exhaustive. There were, for example, some siblings (though comparatively few) who maintained relatively unstressful relationships with their head-injured sister or brother although, except in the two families in which recovery from the head injury had been the greatest, the nature of the relationship was considerably changed.

It can be seen that, for families such as these, the situation can become very complex. Siblings are affected by the accident itself, by the interplay of reactions and relationships between other members of the family, by the changes in personality and abilities of the injured sister or brother. The familiar relationships that once existed between sisters and brothers, however close or distant they were before, have to be renegotiated. In many cases siblings have a number of self-contradictory emotions with regard to their head injured sister or brother, and find it very difficult to tread a consistent path through the minefield of the newly developing relationship. All of them would have benefited from the presence of someone to listen to them and to talk to them from the very beginning, so that the fears and guilts and rejections could have been brought up naturally, as they arose. It is also clear that much of the suffering that families experienced would have been eased, to a greater or lesser extent, by the provision of more information about what to expect, and some degree of training to deal with what can be an extremely difficult and often distressing situation for everyone, not least for the young person at the centre of the web of relationships.

4 Life at home: sources of support

It has been seen in Chapter Two that the families feel very much on their own when they take over responsibility from the hospital or rehabilitation unit. Some families need very little support, others a great deal, but this latter group do not always appear to be the ones who have been the most fortunate in the amount of help that they get. There are a variety of factors that are relevant here, ranging from sheer luck in terms of the level of services provided by a specific Health Authority, to the nature and context of the particular problems experienced by the young people and their families. Two families, living in one of the Health Districts, were given continuing advice and support (see especially the White family, Chapter One).

An additional problem for some families was the geographical area in which they lived. There were problems involved in transport to rehabilitation or day centres; lack of coordination between hospitals in different Health Districts, between Health and Social Service departments, and between Social Service Departments in different areas. The resulting confusion added considerably to the stress that families were under. As one mother said: 'it was outrageous, we were stressed out of our eyeballs'.

Most families were given some help in finding somewhere for their son or daughter to go during the day - to day centres or workshops for disabled people, or they were helped to return to work (but see below). However, when the initial help from the hospital wears off, and the situation at home has returned, as far as the services are concerned, to some sort of 'normal' daily life, the families are often left in circumstances which to them are far from normal, and a daily life that bears little resemblance to the life they led before. As one mother said:

> If he was still in a wheelchair, couldn't speak, incontinent, with one arm, he'd be fine, there'd be lots of help and all sorts of things would happen for him, but he's fallen out of that category; he still can't be left alone

> and so on, but the health service have lost interest - it's quite clear that he now is a very unimportant kind of person because he's better, as far as they're concerned.

In many cases, although physical disabilities may be minor, they are sufficient to make daily life laboured and stressful. One parent repeatedly asked for a hand rail on the bath, because her son tended to slip down in the water, and for a rail on the sloping path up to the front door, because he kept falling down, but neither has been provided. This family has now stopped bothering to ask for help of any kind.

Some families had relatives outside the household who provided moral support, especially the mother's mother and sisters. In most families there was little that they could do in practical terms, and they were as inexperienced as the family itself in the effects that severe head injury could have. In a few families a relative also gave practical help (see below).

'It's a situation where there's no targets'

There are various kinds of help and support that families need when they bring their son or daughter home from the hospital. In families in which the young person concerned needs practical, medical care this was usually forthcoming, at least in the first few months. One of the families that received the most practical help at first is the Bell family (and see Chapter Three). Stephie was seriously injured in a car crash, and is the most physically disabled of the young people in this study, still being unable to walk or to say more than a few words. At first when she came home she was visited twice a week by physiotherapists, by an occupational therapist weekly (who also provided a wheelchair), a district nurse and a speech therapist. Stephie was also attending the local Headway day centre. The family had not been offered any counselling, but Stephie's mother says she, at least, does not need it: 'If I'm going to get over something I'll get over it in my own time. I don't think all the talking in the world changes anything'.

Although very supportive at first, the services began to drop away quite quickly, although the level of need seemed to be much the same. The speech therapist did not come for nearly eight months, and although the family tried to get Stephie to talk this was not giving her the specialist help that she needed. Her mother said: 'in my eyes they know what she needs more than we do, we're not qualified speech therapists are we?'

Although Stephie continued to have a catheter she was not visited by a nurse except when she pulled it out. Her mother continued to wash and dress her and heave her about, although she herself had long-standing back trouble. She was helped by one of her daughters, and also by her own mother, who was of immense practical help in looking after Stephie - in contrast to Mr Bell's mother, who told them that they should have Stephie 'put away'. The only professional who visited was the social worker from the hospital, once a month, and Social Services gave them a grant to build an extension for Stephie. The Bells believed that the doctors had really thought that they would not stick it out, and had expected Stephie back in hospital, but they had underestimated her mother's determination. However, it took its toll - Mrs Bell had to be given various sorts of medication for depression and for panic attacks. She and her husband felt that they never saw each other alone any more, and that their life had reverted to the way it was a few years earlier, before their youngest child left school. Both of them felt very bitter about this:

> We get angry with the situation for the simple reason it took us until my youngest was sixteen to start having a life of our own, and now it's gone again...that's why I feel bitter, that's what I think they've taken away from us. Because we've worked hard for these things, you know, since day one, and now we're back to square one again.

Stephie continued to go to Headway twice a week, and she began to attend a private rehabilitation centre for an hour or so a few times a week, paid for out of an interim payment from the compensation:

> They filled us in on what has to be done, and it's got to be done in the very near future, that's for her hands and legs and what have you...whatever it is, it's going to be a long, long drawn out thing, I mean I feel it's a situation where there's no targets, you cannot say well in six months time you're going to walk.

The Bells were relieved that something was going to be done about Stephie, but surprised that the further treatment which is now said to be vital for her recovery only appeared to become available when they were in a position to pay for it.

'He's a prisoner in his own home'

Once their son or daughter has come home, and after the initial links with the rehabilitation unit have been severed, many families feel that they are just forgotten. One young man, Alec Robinson, said 'I feel like I've been dumped'. Two years after his accident he still feels that he needs physiotherapy for his arm and leg, which are partly paralysed. In addition to the head injury, Alec also suffered a severe leg injury in his accident, almost severing it. He last saw a physiotherapist a year ago, but has not seen a doctor for much longer. His mother said:

> I'm quite mad really that he hasn't had a proper check up with the doctor, to check his leg. His leg always worries him, he seems to think that one day it's going to fall off, that the wire at the side is going to break and it's going to fall off, and no matter what I say, you can't convince him, but I still think that he should have a proper check up with a consultant.

His parents also feel that he should also see a neurologist, because he has not seen one since he left hospital:

> The day we left the hospital [eighteen months ago] I said to the doctor 'is there anything that we should be doing,' you know, we were worried, we've never come across head injuries before, we didn't know whether he still had the clot, what had happened or nothing, they never explained nothing to us and he said, 'no nothing' - you know, goodbye and good luck, nothing. I think when he first came home I was frightened more than anything; he couldn't walk...we didn't really know much about head injuries, nobody ever really sat down and explained what would happen when he left hospital, and the first few months he was home, we were worried: what if he falls? What if he hits his head? To this day we've not been told anything although it's been two years, you know, you *still* worry all the time.

One of the problems is that the results of a head injury may continue indefinitely. There may be good periods, but these may well be followed by bad ones. Things may go smoothly for a bit, and then another crisis will arise. By following the lives of these families over a year or so it has been possible to document the ups and downs from month to month. Alec's mother, for example, said at one point that 'the family is pretty much back to normal', but six months later she said: 'I said to you before that we felt that everything was almost as back to normal as it is going to be, but all of a sudden... everything had flared up, and got us all down'. Among other things, Alec was having a great deal of trouble with his leg 'he takes a lot of pain killers, it's getting worse, a lot worse'. Alec and his parents felt that he needed physiotherapy, so they contacted a social worker to try to organize it:

> We're still toing and froing, the social worker's trying to work something out, nobody knows what's going on. He's supposed to be having physiotherapy, but nobody seems to know much about that. The doctor doesn't know anything about it, the hospital where he used to go doesn't...so at the moment nobody knows what's going on, it's a bit confusing, but the social worker's trying to work it out.

Alec left the 'college course' he had been on, which seemed to him to consist mainly of sweeping up or weeding. With help from his parents and the social worker he moved out of the family home and gave up going to college. He spent the days indoors watching television, and the evenings getting drunk. In spite of his physical problems, he had his application for a mobility allowance turned down. Alec was having difficulty walking to the corner shop, especially carrying something, because of his bad arm, and his leg very quickly started dragging. The social worker, in spite of her efforts to help, was now considered, at least by Alec's father, to be 'dead useless':

> She hasn't taken any interest in him whatsoever. He's been turned down for mobility allowance, twice. Nobody in the mobility department has ever been to see him or nothing. He's had a letter to say he's not disabled, he's not entitled to mobility allowance; then we had a letter saying that we've got to go to a tribunal - that was four months ago and nobody's bothered, nobody is interested in him whatsoever.

Alec's father is saddened by the meagre quality of the life his son lives:

> He's a prisoner in his own home, he can't go out...he can't get on the bus, he can't carry nothing, what can he do? I mean, the other day I was bloody near in tears - he was trying to struggle back from the shop with a carrier bag...and he just spilt it on the ground, and he lost all the shopping; but he *wants* to go up there on his own, the shop is just up the road but to get there and back again takes him about three quarters of an hour - and they say he's not disabled. He gets very frustrated with himself.

In spite of the fact that Alec has a social worker, he and his father are still confused about what is happening. His parents commented that the hospital treatment, when he was an in-patient, was 'unbeatable anywhere in the world', but that after he came home the communication and support had been minimal.

'There are no guidelines'

Dean Marshall came home from hospital his mother was told that he would be able to attend a day centre five days a week, and that he would continue to have regular occupational therapy sessions. He was also promised psychological help, because he was having violent mood swings, and his mother was assured that he would be called back to the rehabilitation unit to see how things were going in three weeks time. None of these things came about. He was offered two days a week at a Headway Centre, and no occupational therapy or psychological help was arranged for him: 'We were given a lot of assurances which never came to fruition. There's been nothing, no one came near us'. Part of the problem was not only that the family live at a considerable distance outside the catchment area of the hospital in which Dean had been an in-patient, but also that they live on the border of two counties, resulting in confusion about which Health District and which Social Services Department should be involved. The family felt themselves to be in a nomansland, in which no one, including the service providers themselves, seemed to know who was responsible for the provision of services to Dean. Struggling through the maze, Mrs Marshall finally managed to arrange some occupational therapy for him. The only person who came to the house was someone to assess whether the house was safe for Dean, but she was not the sort of person that Mrs Marshall felt she could talk to: 'She gave me information that was wrong anyway, I felt that probably if she wanted to sit and chat to me she'd learn more from me than I'd learn from her'. Mrs Marshall had assumed that Dean's problems would be sorted out when they went for their appointment at the hospital three weeks after he came home. In the event, it was not three weeks but four months before they were given an appointment.

> We got to the stage where we just felt totally abandoned. One of the big frustrations is the real lack of somebody to advise us. There are no guidelines. I would have liked, right at the very start, somebody actually sitting down with us and saying, you know it's going to be a really long hard road ahead and there are these organisations and these people that could help and advise you - not just leave you to your own devices. We should have been in touch with a social worker at the hospital, but I didn't even know one existed, it was only through sheer frustration that I got hold of one locally - it took us five weeks to get hold of her...we never had a thing, not a thing.

The constant strain at home affected the relationship between Dean's mother and her fiance. He was trying very hard to be supportive, but found the situation hard to cope with, mainly because of the constant demands that Dean made on their time and energy ('our time together has changed' he said sadly). At one point the relationship almost broke down altogether because, as Mrs Marshall pointed out to her fiance: 'I don't need problems with you, I need support; I'm not getting it from anywhere else'.

Apart from the practical help that was lacking, Dean's offensiveness towards his mother was a major problem:

> We felt that he ought to be seeing a psychiatrist. We don't think he's mad or anything, but somebody that he can talk to that's going to

understand, and try and help him...we don't even know if there is such a person, we don't even know where to find him and we feel that now if we went and spoke to them, whoever it is, they would probably turn round and say, 'well what are you talking to me for?'

In a roundabout way this family eventually found someone who could help them with some of their problems. They were put in touch with the Disabilities Initiative Centre, and Mrs Marshall said that one member of staff there was 'fantastic, she really was, I felt I could talk to her and she understood some of the things I was going through'.

In spite of this source of help, life continued to be a struggle to return to some semblance of normality:

> You learn to take it in your stride but you are uptight, you are worn out, you are emotionally strained anyway...and then you're fighting the system, fighting everybody the whole of the time.

Fourteen months after Dean's accident, his mother said:

> All I want to do is to get his life back in order and in turn put our life back in order. I mean, it was totally turned upside down and I suppose since then we've adapted and gone on and progressed, but we're not finished with anything...there's still more to go and more things to do. I feel we are all on hold, as though we're going through the motions but sort of not moving forward at all. We just seem to have come to a dead end.

Sixteen months later she still felt that little had been resolved, but by this time had come to realise that there was probably never going to be a time when she could feel that Dean's life was on an even keel: 'the problems are always going to be there'.

'I'm not here to answer your questions'

One family felt strongly that their son should have had a check up since he left rehabilitation. He had been very severely injured in an accident in which he had been assumed dead. Although he has made what appears to be the most successful return to family and work environment of all the young people in the study, and his personality perhaps the least affected of all of them, his short term memory is still said to be 'diabolical', his balance is not perfect and his eyes are slightly 'glazed'.

Their son had been told originally by a doctor at the hospital that 'he has got less brain cells so he really shouldn't drink like a normal person'. These odd bits of information, whether or not they were given in a sensible context, are not exactly helpful, and simply add to the confusion that many families feel. What does it mean to say that someone has 'less brain cells'? How many brain cells does someone have? What is a 'normal' person? What does a 'normal person' drink? It is hardly surprising that no one knows how much care they should take. In this family, lack of sufficient advice or guidance meant that the son felt confident enough to join in sporting activities which risked serious damage to his head.

His parents, a year after his accident, were very keen for him to have a neurological check up, and some routine tests, and insisted on an appointment with the neurologist, but when they did see him they came away disappointed:

> It consisted of about five minutes in the consultant's surgery, standing on one leg and then the other and then he pricked you with a pin in a few places - and talk about *rude*: 'well, I wouldn't have called you back,' he said, 'and I'm not here to answer your questions. All I will say is, having seen him again now, he's making a remarkable recovery, quite beyond what was expected.'

These parents knew that already, but this was not their point. They had expected more detailed tests, as he had had before, and some information and guidance about what he should or should not do.

Not all consultants were so unhelpful. There is one, in particular, whom all the young people felt had been very helpful, although visits to him were very short, and few and far between. This consultant seemed to understand the emotions and problems that almost inevitably seem to follow in the wake of severe head injuries. This was a comfort, because it made people feel that what was happening to them was expected, but there was very seldom anything tangible offered in the way of help to make things easier to get through the long period of recovery. This consultant, whom the young people described as understanding, was seldom actually seen, and almost impossible to get hold of, thus the parents were rather less positive about him. Many of the families felt that the consultant and rehabilitation team, although they were seen to have done an enormous amount for their patients while they were in the hospital, had relinquished their responsibility once the head injured person had gone home, with no established structure in place to continue providing the necessary support.

This lack of support was most obvious in relation to families who were already isolated from the world of the professionals. In these cases there seems to be little attempt by the latter to establish effective communication, in spite of the evident need for help. Such families tend to feel that nobody at all cares what happens to them, and each rejection that they encounter increases their sense of isolation. It is quite possible that the professionals consider such families awkward and difficult to please, but from the families' point of view they are simply not getting the kind of support they so obviously need. In one case, for example, the head injured young man had already made several serious suicide attempts, and his parents believed that he might well try again. They were told that psychiatric help would be arranged for him, but when it failed to materialize they withdrew into their own world, and are very unlikely to seek further help. Now, whenever their son goes out, they half-expect to see a policeman on the doorstep, saying 'I'm sorry, it's your son...'.

'You're the first person that has ever listened'

One of the most necessary services that was missing for most families was someone to talk to who was experienced in head injury and its consequences, whether medical, intellectual, behavioural or social. In the first few months after returning home, most families had access to a social worker attached to the hospital, and they were invaluable sources of help for filling in forms for allowances, and other practical things that had to be done. Later, however, if they could get social workers, they tended not be specialists in head injury, and thus could not provide the kind of help that families began to need, as one parent said: 'He listens, but that's more or less all he does. You can talk to him as much as you like but he doesn't give you the guidance which really you need'.

Listening was an important function, however, even without specialist knowledge, or the ability to help, and usually there was no one who automatically took on this listening role. In one instance, for example, in an interview with a young man and his parents which was fraught with tension and hostility, the son said:

> You are the first person Mum and Dad have put across [anything] to and you're the first person that has ever listened to them about what trouble they've had.

In another family, after the first interview with the parents and their son, the mother said:

> Come back whenever you like, you're very welcome because actually it's good for us to talk to somebody, to get it out of one's system...I think I would have liked somebody like you right from the word go. Somebody who is not involved in it...because you don't have that support in

hospital. We'd have been able to take a rational view then - we were quite irrational really at times.

In one area, a Care Manager was provided from the very beginning, and to the White family she was an invaluable source of advice and encouragement. Although she has recently retired, and a replacement has taken over her role, she has remained a true friend:

> She said, 'I'll be there if you ever need me, if ever you want to pick the phone up, I'll be there.' She doesn't just come to see Colin, she's concerned if the rest of us need any sort of boosting up anywhere along the line...All I feel is if anything really awful reared it's head there'd be somebody who knew all about this, and I wouldn't have to repeat the whole thing right over to somebody totally out of the blue that I didn't know - it's like having an old friend really isn't it? It's a lot easier if somebody knows what you've been through. I do think that there should be ways of somebody to be able to just sort of say I can talk to so and so, and they won't mind if I'm upset.

The Whites were lucky; the Care Manager not only was a specialist in head injury, but also visited the family in their own home, so that the situation was very informal, and the whole family could interact naturally. For another parent, however, in a different area, it not only took a long time to get referred to a counsellor by a G.P., but the circumstances of the counselling was very artificial:

> I wasn't really comfortable with it, if I'm really honest, everything was too twee. It was supposed to look comfortable and it was all too perfect - almost to the point of intimidation, if you know what I mean. It was all too perfect, it was all set up.

However, it confirmed the view of this mother that to be able to sit and talk to someone would have been useful from the beginning. Ideally, however, this should not have to take place in a specially created counselling environment, with a box of tissues strategically placed within reach, but at home, over a cup of coffee.

For another family, there was no apparent source of counselling:

> One of my greatest kind of sadnesses about the system that we have is in terms of what the health service could have done for him - provide him with some therapy, as *essential* From the day he was in hospital, if he could have had a kind of counsellor-therapist, building up a relationship all this time, which would help him through lots of the things, quite independent of us...that is for me one of the greatest omissions, and now of course it's really difficult to pick up.

The search for identity is a recurring theme, and something that some parents feel could be helped by counselling or therapy:

> He's really searching for himself, and it feels like that is just not catered for at all, although he's had a head injury, and therefore that would be considered, in my view, to be something that was necessary, and it isn't around, it just isn't.

'He said "I can tell you what's happening"'

One invaluable source of practical help and advice that was identified by a number of families was their local Headway centre. Headway (the National Head Injuries Association) is a registered charity, and Headway groups have been set up all over the country to give advice and support to head injured people and their families. Some run day centres, and others consist mainly of evening discussion groups.

Three families were living too far away from any Headway to be able to attend evening meetings, or go to a Headway centre. Seven young people spent some time at their local Headway day centre, six at the same one. All six of these, and their families, were full of praise for the centre and, in particular, for the man who runs it. This particular centre provides three important functions. First, it provides occupation and training during the day, with continuous supervision and stimulus, thus allowing the possibility of very real progress. Second, there are monthly evening meetings either with an invited speaker, or just to talk over coffee. Third, the person in charge, J.D., is one of the very few people available to the young people and their families, who is not only prepared to listen, but also to give straightforward and practical advice. Parents can telephone him in despair as the situation at home spirals towards disaster, and get down to earth advice, as well as being invited to come and talk it over - with or without their head injured son or daughter, or other members of the family.

One of the parents rang J.D. at a point when her son's control over the lives of everyone in the household had taken hold, to the extent that he expected everyone to give into him, and quickly became aggressive if he was thwarted. J.D. listened at length to this parent, and then told her what had gone wrong:

> He said 'I can tell you what's happening,' and everything he said was right, he'd *got* it. He said, 'this is what's happening isn't it? Basically I'm going to tell you what you've done wrong. You have run round behind him, you've cossetted him, you've done this for him, you've done that for him...you've babied him'. Everything he said, I said, 'yes,

> you're right.' He said, 'it's natural what you've done, but you've done too much now, and he's taking advantage'. I've got into a situation that I can't handle now...and he gets drunk at least three times a week, his mates think it's funny, but then J.D. said 'yes,they think it's funny and this is why they take him out, they're really taking the mickey out of him.'

This was the first time in two and a half years that anyone had told this mother what she should or should not be doing, in spite of the fact that the psychologist from the hospital where her son had been for rehabilitation had seen him off and on during most of that period, in connection with his return to work. Another parent said:

> He was super, I could have chatted for hours. He will let you shout at him over the telephone and he'll take you through a few things and then he'll get somebody to ring you that's actually gone through it. They will talk you through it...that was a great comfort and I thought, well yes, there is hope. It's all right people saying to you, 'oh he'll be all right, he'll be all right' and you think, you don't know what you're talking about. But to actually speak to somebody that had a head injury - and I thought, oh, they sound normal!

This family lived some distance from Headway, but as a result of their contact with J.D. they and a group of local people who had been head injured, and families, set up a local Headway group (see below).

Not only their parents, but also the head injured people can turn to him for advice and support independently. One boy said approvingly 'He's all right, he's there for the people'. Coming from him, this was high praise. Another young man praised the day centre there: 'It was brilliant because it gave me back everything socially, and working, and doing different things'. He stopped going for a bit, because he felt he wanted to 'go on from there', but he went back later to help them with some building work. This increased his self-confidence because he could be justly proud of the work he had done. At this stage he said that when he looked at the other people there he thought how lucky he was. Headway, for him, was an important part of his rehabilitation, as it is for many others.

'He felt that he was being branded'

Not all the young people wanted to go to Headway. Six rejected it because they felt that the people there were 'disabled' and that they themselves were not, or at least not to the same extent. However, it was not always possible to distinguish the reactions of the parents from those of the young people themselves. One father, for example, said:

> When I saw what was down there, I said, 'no way.' [The social worker] took him down there and he was upset. And he said, 'I'm not going there again'. His big fear was that if he became an epileptic or his recovery started to reverse that he could end up like some of these people. I mean he was getting mixed up with people that never fully recovered from brain tumours and what have you, and that's what I said, he should have been counselled on that, not just taken down to Headway...the nearest bloke to his age was in his thirties, and most of them were strokes and brain tumours. He felt that he was being branded, you know, 'that's your category there' and that was his great fear.

His son agreed: 'Oh that place frightened me' he said; and another said: 'I saw three people in wheelchairs sat there and I thought, no'. One young man who also went to have a look at the local Headway centre, rejected the idea of going there (or to any other day centre):

> They're a waste of time for my sort. They're just somewhere to go, it's like gaol sort of thing. They're crap. I spend most of my time going down the pub. I get so bored.

His mother said the same thing, slightly differently, and it is hard to know, in this instance, who really initiated the attitude towards Headway:

> To tell you the truth it just wasn't his cup of tea, I think we can honestly say that we are very fortunate in having him the way he is, and this might sound awful but he probably don't see himself - well, he's not as bad as what they were and he just couldn't handle it and quite honestly I couldn't.

Three of the families in the study were part of a group who set up a new Headway in another town. At present this meets as a discussion group, with some social occasions, but there is no day centre. It is backed by the local consultant in rehabilitation, who gives members his support and advice. The Headway environment was seen as a safe context in which to bare one's soul, as one mother said:

> They can all say things without feeling embarrassed, or worried that a confidence will be betrayed because they've all more or less been somewhere along the line. I always come out of there thinking I'm glad I went; I think it's because nobody puts a front up and because everybody feels safe.

'It's just lack of confidence'

Only three of the twenty young people have returned to a life situation that is similar to the one they were in before their accident, one working full time, and the other two as students. Of the rest, six are attending day centres or workshops for people with disabilities, one is at a residential college, two work part-time (unpaid) and nine are not doing anything. Of these nine two are still very dependent on their families, but may move on to attending day centres. Four were taken back into their old jobs, or apprenticeship courses, with the expectation, at least in three cases, that the unpaid phase would develop into normal paid employment. None of these jobs lasted. The problems faced by one of these young people, Sam Green, has been discussed above (Chapter Two). Another of those who returned to their previous workplace was Craig Brown, and to begin with things went well. When he started, eight months after his discharge from hospital, his mother said:

> They really are a caring company...he's back there now. [the psychologist] is gradually working him into the job. She's been doing this over a period of about three months. He's on three whole days now and two afternoons. She laid down some rules which the firm has to stick by; he loves his job and he's good at it...they're keeping him on disability benefit until they feel he can take the stress of a full-time job.

Five months later, he was still at work, but still not being paid:

> He's still on disability benefit, which upsets him a lot, it gets him quite angry, but I can tell you honestly I don't think he's fit to go back - he gets angry when I say it...this week he had an incident, he was told to use the band saw, which is a big saw, and his words were: 'I freaked out, I couldn't use it.' He got somebody else to do it for him, and they're all very friendly and very helpful, but it's still there, it's just lack of confidence. He loses his temper very, very quickly. He's been told to watch it apparently. He's very volatile.

Three months later he was still not being paid for his work, and this was upsetting him:

> They haven't taken Craig back to work. They keep telling me there's nothing wrong with his work, he does his job well, they're pleased with what he does. Now that boy is working apparently full time there, and is still on £51 a week benefit, I feel they're using him, every time that boy says 'my certificate runs out next Monday' it's 'oh well we'll talk to you

> about it before your certificate runs out,' or 'We will take you back', 'oh, we've just got to see the accountant about you.' That boy is getting so screwed up and frustrated now, because he's written down all the hours that he's done for them for nothing, it's about 900 hours. He's getting very frustrated and we're getting it at home.

Two months later all seemed to be well. His mother had rung up the psychologist who had set the work up for him after his head injury, and made 'a bit of a fuss'. As a result, Craig was put back on the payroll. Within a few weeks, however, Craig was told that he was being 'laid off'. He was then back at home all day, doing nothing. He went to his mother one day in tears, and said that perhaps his firm had kept him on after his accident because they felt they had to, and they knew that he was not quite '100 per cent' His mother said that '*he* knows he is not quite 100 per cent' and that he now seems to be getting worse:

> He's regressing a bit, especially in the mornings, it takes a little longer to come round. Once he's come round, he isn't too bad now - well, he doesn't walk straight. But perhaps he's been back to work long enough for people to figure out that he's not quite the same person.

At home he became restless and irritable. His mother felt she could not go back to the life that they had led for so long following Craig's accident:

> I thought, oh Christ, I can't stand this again, I can't cope with this. I said, 'look Craig, I'll give you three months to get a job and then you can clear off, you can go this time, you can go out there in this big wide world and find out what it's all about; until you've been out there, you don't know how hard it is if you're not satisfied here.

Craig did manage to get a temporary job, for a few weeks, which eased the situation, but in the long term there is probably going to be further frustration and resulting upheavals at home. It is quite probable that the 'caring' employers who took him back so soon after his accident were doing it for Craig's benefit, and that they fully expected to be able to take him on the payroll again. For a period, at least, Craig's sense of self worth increased, but the let-down was all the greater in the end, not only because of his raised hopes, but also because he had to face again the fact that he was not fully recovered from the effects of his head injury. The setting up of the job, done as it was by the psychologist from the hospital, was as near to ideal as it could have been, but there was a lack of communication somewhere. Craig's employer should have been able to tell Craig what the problems were with his work, instead of appearing to string him along and actually put him on the payroll, and then 'lay him off' almost immediately. In another instance, a young man who had been a bricklayer for eight years before his accident, went out on to the site and found that he had lost all his 'speed and confidence', and after his retraining period was not taken onto the payroll.

The experiences of these young men highlight a number of problems. If people with head injuries are to be able to return to work there are various criteria that must be satisfied. It is no good going back to work unless there is going to be continuous monitoring of the situation. The work that a head injured person is given must be something he (or she) can actually do, so that 'speed and confidence' have a chance to develop, and the environment should be a supportive one, in which lack of confidence and frustration can be met with patience and understanding. Getting back to work is often a significant step towards the recovery of self esteem, as one young man says: 'I want to get out into the big bad world and make my own bucks rather than going down the post office every Wednesday and cashing my giro. I feel a right dosser'.

For most of the young people and their families the main problem that they faced in the enduring aftermath of a severe head injury was the lack of adequate information, advice and support. As has been seen in this and earlier chapters, life at home may be totally disrupted, and only one family out of the fifteen in which the head injured person is still currently living at home, could be said to be in a stable equilibrium, and the members of the family at peace with themselves. Perhaps the most needed of all services is counselling. As one parent said, one of his greatest sadnesses about the National Health Service was that there was nobody there from the very beginning, when the person who had suffered a severe head injury first came out of a coma:

> If he could have had a kind of counsellor-therapist, building up a relationship all this time, which would have helped him through lots of the things, quite independent of us. That is for me one of the greatest omissions, and now of course it's really difficult to pick up.

Similarly, as has been shown, parents and siblings often need someone to talk to from the very beginning. In some cases a social worker adopted this role in the hospital, but the relationship was not often continued for long, if at all, when the person moved away, or went home. Once back in the home environment, access to local social workers was seldom a problem, and these were invaluable in the context of practical issues. They arranged daytime activities, helped to fill in the long and complicated forms that had to be filled in for allowances, and generally tried to sort out practical problems. In many cases, however, the social workers had not had a great deal of experience with head injured people and their families. Thus they were often unable to respond to the more complex individual and familial problems that developed in the months, and even years, after the severe head injury.

5 Friends

In many cases, the friends that were around before the accident begin to drop away quite soon afterwards. Often their first reaction was to crowd around the hospital bed, but as the weeks and months passed over half of the young people found that their friends seemed to melt away. The reasons for this are often complex. For one thing, as has been seen, coming home after a severe head injury does not mean that someone can immediately jump back into the life that they had led before. The person may still be very house bound, and at the very least may have been advised by doctors not to stay up late at night and not to drink alcohol, thus parents may feel that they have to limit outside activities quite severely. For some of the young men, particularly, normal activities with their friends had tended to be centred round the pub, or, to put it round the other way, the group who met and drank in the pub were seen as friends. If someone was unable to join in the activity, then the friendship frequently lapsed. Allan (1979) refers to this as 'mateship' as opposed to 'friendship', which he suggests is appropriate to more personal relationships. Of course, by no means all of the people who were considered friends were only drinking companions. Many relationships that had been close friendships also crumbled in the aftermath of these accidents.

Sometimes friends are frightened off by parents at an early stage. One father, devastated by what had happened to his son, turned on the boy's friends when they visited the hospital, as his sister describes:

> Dad just frightened them off, sort of said well this is what happens if you do so and so, you know, if you're silly, and they were so embarrassed, they were all cringing and I was cringing; mum and dad should have gone away, let his friends talk to him, see him, do what ever they wanted, but they didn't, they stayed there and dad was quite nasty. Perhaps his friends don't want to be in that situation again.

Some found that their friends just gradually withdrew. As one mother said with regard to her son, who now spends all his time sitting at home: 'His old mates don't want to know him anymore...they just stopped bothering with him'. Another young man, who had had many friends before his accident, was left with one good friend, but even this one had begun to pull out of the relationship. He did not do it in a straightforward manner, but constantly backed out of arrangements that had been made: 'he'll make promises that he's coming over and then it's "Oh, sorry, I can't make it"'. Similar situations were reported in other families. One woman said that when her son was first in hospital lots of his friends came to visit him:

> When it first happened they were all up the hospital, now they come up occasionally; they've worn off now, you only get the odd one come in and I think it's when it's pouring with rain and there's nothing to do.

This happened in other cases; one mother said that her son's friends soon disappeared: 'they never bothered to come, he wasn't one of the boys any more, was he? All that changed'.

It is perhaps understandable that the friends of these young people, even if they survive the emotional turmoil and perhaps quite violent stages of recovery, continue to feel some awkwardness with them. Often they have changed quite dramatically in the things they can or cannot do, or in their range of interests. Others are also changed in personality, and it is perhaps this aspect that makes it hard for other people, not only their peers, to re-establish rapport. Members of the families face the same problems, but in most cases, though not in all, they are prepared to renegotiate their relationships (see above). Many of the young friends, however, are reluctant to take this on. It is also relevant in this situation that a significant period of time has often elapsed since they were active friends together. During that time all of them are one or two years older, their activities may have changed, and their individual preoccupations led them on diverging paths.

'I have no history'

It is not only the practical aspects of the relationship between friends that is relevant here. It is clear that in many cases the very nature and quality of the relationship between the young person and his or her former friends has changed. The person who has had a severe head injury often comes home from hospital feeling and behaving differently from before the accident. To their friends they may appear to be quite changed, different people altogether in some quite fundamental ways. It is significant that those young people in the study who retained their friends, and related to them in much the same way as before, are those who are the least changed in themselves.

In some cases it is the head injured person him or herself who does not want to take up with old friends, preferring to make new friends who are unaware of what has happened, or at least are unaware of any changes that have taken place. New friends cannot make comparisons with what someone was like before - what a person is like now is, as far as they are concerned, what he or she has always been like. Thus it is possible for the people who have suffered a head injury, and who are nervous and unsure of their own identity, to be accepted for what they are. Jenny Cooper, for example, has not only found that her old friends have moved on to do new things in different places, but she also prefers to spend her time with people she has got to know since her accident. Jenny is very aware that she has changed, but because she cannot remember exactly what she was like she is worried that these changes are for the worse, and that her old friends will see this. She says 'I don't know my history, I have no history', and reads her old diaries to try to discover her old self. All she can say at the moment is that she wants to get back to normal though 'its hard for me to say "normal" because I can't really remember how I was before...I know I was a lot happier before'. For a period of time, before she returned to the academic environment which she had been part of before, she chose to have a boyfriend who was quite outside her own social circle:

> I think it's easier for her to go out with someone like that, she probably feels that she can relate to him better, because he hasn't been through college and because she's not expected to keep up. I think she finds it easier to make new friends, who didn't know her beforehand, so it's easier to sort of cover up the gaps.

Matt Lewis, like Jenny, was also searching for his identity. By showing his friends things that had belonged to him before his accident, and that were still his now, he would try to establish a continuum from the past to the present:

> His behaviour with his friends is very egocentric and he seems to be searching for himself because what he will do...is to go to his room with them and turn his room out and say 'this is my book I had when I was at school and this is mine, this is mine,' it's like his identity is in his belongings and he's searching, trying to show them.

In Matt's case, his friends are willing to visit him, even though the relationship has changed dramatically. They believe that he will return to how he was before, and are prepared to stay around in the meantime. In that sense he is more fortunate than many others in the study.

Philip Brent had less understanding friends. When he was first in hospital there were many friends round his bed, but now he only had one left, who had stuck with him through his long recovery, including a 'violent' stage. Philip still sees his other old friends occasionally, when his friend Bob takes him over to the pub, but the nature of the relationships have changed:

> They treat him differently, like they would a child. They ask Bob questions about Philip, instead of asking Philip the questions direct - which makes him very angry.

Philip's parents say his friends are 'useless', and seem to try to put him off wanting to see them. It is hard to know how far this is because it upsets them to see him humiliated by them, and how much it is done in order to keep him at home under their eagle eyes. Philip himself feels that he is very changed now, because he no longer wants to live the life he used to - drinking and smoking and larking about:

> I'm not like that anymore...and the thing is that people that knew me before they - well, not disowned me, but they avoid me, they don't really associate with me now, I don't know why, they probably think I'm mad or something.

In fact he now says he does not like his friends any more anyway. He says that they are 'stupid' and implies that they are also smug because they are all right and he is not: 'They all think they are perfect and nothing is going to happen to them, and I just think, yes, you wait, it will happen'.

There are others who have simply lost the desire to go out with friends; some have become rather solitary and in some cases unaware of themselves as part of a social environment. One mother describes her son in quite harsh terms:

> His social skills are almost non-existent; he did let himself go rather and it was a case of just getting him to look at himself, I mean, I still don't think he knows himself. He's very lonely. There's been definitely a change of character, and he's lost a lot of friends.

'They get him paralytic'

Some of the young people, on the other hand, are keen to retain their friends, and to return to normal activities outside the home, especially in the evenings. Often these 'normal activities' involved heavy drinking, which they were advised against when they left hospital, thus parents would try to prevent their children going out with their drinking friends. This protective behaviour sometimes drove away old friends, or made it too embarrassing for their son or daughter to continue the friendship, as one father admitted:

> What used to happen is whenever anyone called for him to go out I'd say, 'well you know that Roy isn't allowed at do this and isn't allowed to do that.' And they'd say, 'yes that's fine.' And I'd say, 'well in a way that's making you responsible. You are aware of that?'

The burden of taking responsibility for him drove many of Roy's old friends to view him as an unsatisfactory drinking partner, and to let him go. Roy resented this, but he also, in some ways, preferred (as Jenny Cooper did) to find new friends who did not know what he had been like before, and thus did not make him feel 'inferior'. His father would also buttonhole his new friends and tell them about the head injury and what Roy should not do, so Roy would arrange to meet them away from the house. He continued to drink and would come home almost unable to walk, and 'crash out' at once. His parents tried to stop him, for his own good:

> We've got to be very cruel to Roy sometimes, and when he says, 'well why can't I do this, why can't I go out all night with my friends? why can't I be like other people?' I've got to be very cruel to him and I'll say 'Roy, you are *not* like other people, you've just got to wait a bit'...and then he'll argue. It's trying to bring Roy down to earth but it's the cruelest thing to do to say they're not the same as others isn't it?

Other parents found themselves in similar situations. Their sons wanted to go out and live the life they had led before their head injury:

> He's got a lot of mates at the moment that are taking him out, he's twenty-one years old this year and he's now behaving like a fourteen year old, he gets out with his mates and they get him paralytic, and some of his mates, honest to god, they're undesirable...he's still drinking like a fish and he gets drunk very quickly.

'People think you're being anti-social'

One very significant problem in the preservation of old friendships, and the making of new ones, is that almost all the head injured people are extremely low in self confidence. This often makes ordinary social occasions difficult to deal with, and sometimes leads to problems. This lack of confidence is described by one:

> I was in a good job, had a good social life, got on with everyone, most of that has been taken away. It's building it up again yourself. Like some

people don't understand, if they don't start the conversation off, I find it really hard to start off a conversation...people think you're being anti-social but it's really hard, unless someone talks to you.

This lack of confidence seems to be compounded by a nervousness in crowded places, often reported by these young people. The desire to 'get back to normal' by going to the pub and drinking was, in fact, often more an ordeal than a relaxing experience. One young man, Mac, who insisted on going to the pub although he felt very uncomfortable and paranoid among a crowd of people, tended to express this by acting aggressively towards his drinking friends, as his brother said:

Because everybody else was doing just normal stuff, you were just fed up and you would take the piss out of everybody in the pub, you wound them up.

But according to Mac, he was only trying to assert himself:

There are so many assholes who think that because I've had an accident I'm some helpless little wimp. I won't have that anymore. I've had enough of it. I'm not saying I'm going to go and fight someone but I'm just saying if people are going to patronise me and take advantage and stuff, they're going to learn, it's as simple as that. If they're offering violence I'm not going to say, 'no don't pick on me, don't pick on me, I'm only a weak little boy.'

Some of the young people feel that this experience has taught them who their real friends are. One said sadly: 'I don't get on with people now, when I'm in groups of people I'm always the odd one out because I'm the one with a head injury and I'm the one who can't do it'. Another said that he had lost friends because no one really knows what it is like to have a head injury:

No one can fully understand I don't think, not unless you're the person in that situation...like the nurses in the hospital are around them all the time, they know what they're doing and that, but they don't really *know*. Its just, how can you describe it? People don't understand, like, say I'm in a pub and there's something really simple will wind me up, which wouldn't normally wind me up, and people don't understand why I'm doing that. I *look* perfectly normal, I think.

This highlights an important point. As some of these young people say, they are often easily 'wound up' by circumstances that would not have disturbed them before, and because there is nothing to show that they have had a head injury, people who do not know may be surprised, and sometimes angered, by some of their reactions.

'It's never really occurred to him that he's disabled'

Although social relationships may be hard, and physical recovery not always progressing very quickly, few of the young people saw themselves as disabled, and seldom sought friends among the people they met at day centres or 'disabled workshops'. As one put it, he was not disabled, just recovering from an accident. One mother said:

> He doesn't really consider himself disabled...he was upset when the doctor said that he was disabled and that he would always be disabled, I can remember him coming out of the surgery saying 'he just said I was going to be disabled.' And I said, 'well you are aren't you?' 'Oh' he said, 'oh, I suppose I am.' But it's never really occurred to him that he's disabled, and I suppose in a way it's a good thing, you try and live a normal life if you can.

This determination not to be labelled 'disabled' often meant that these young people not only did not want to have friends with disabilities, but also did not want to join in activities specifically for people with disabilities, as one mother said:

> He said 'I don't want to go back to the disabled swimming group, because I don't feel like I'm fitting in there, I'm not really ill enough to be in a disabled group' and I really felt like crying, I mean it was so sad. It's true isn't it, he's not, he doesn't. He needs a group where he's got time given to him but he doesn't need what goes with the group, like the wheelchairs and all, and the frames.

In one case a friendship that developed in the context of a workshop for young people with disabilities was discouraged by the father, who tried to steer his son in a different direction:

> He got friendly with this guy who is in a wheelchair, a very nice bloke, I must admit...but again, you can't turn round and say 'well, look, it's fine having him as a friend, but don't go overboard, because you really should be looking for friendship on the able bodied side'.. [we can] try and push him in other directions, not to say that he forgets about Len, but we rather think that's a good thing.

But for his son, as his life is at the moment, he sees his old friends living in a world which is currently out of his reach:

> All the friends that I had have cars, they go out drinking and really have a good time and go to discos and things like that. Now, me, I can't drink because I'm on pills, I can't drive because I'm epileptic, I can't go to

discos because of my head, I go all dizzy with the music, which does my head in.

His old friends do not understand what he feels like, and he prefers to be with people who have some understanding of him as he is now. He has met someone now who provides the sort of friendship that he needs:

> He's pretty good on computers and I've had some knowledge from him, so I can work on that...it's just really sort of finding things to do things that are not stupid, like going with the venture scouts - they've been wanting me to go abseiling and other things like that. I don't really like running down the side of a building and things like that.

'From then on it was all downhill'

Perhaps the most difficult of all the non-familial relationships, and the most likely to collapse under the strain, are those between girlfriend and boyfriend.

In instances where relationships were well-established before the accident, they tended to survive in the early weeks, or even months, of the head injury, but few continued beyond the critical stages. It is, perhaps, easy to continue to love and care for someone who is in a coma, who is, in a sense, a non-partner in the relationship, or who is still highly dependent in a hospital environment, but it is harder to carry this through into daily life, with all the physical and emotional problems that are part and parcel of the recovery process. Few of the boyfriends and girlfriends, often themselves still in their teenage years, feel committed enough to cope with someone who appears to be very different from the person they were going out with, or even fell in love with, before the accident. One young woman said wistfully about her ex-boyfriend: 'I'd like to say he was a friend now, but I don't really think he's a friend. I think he's trying to keep distant from me...I just think it's all a bit frightening for him'.

It is at this point that parents take over again, continuing or returning to the parental caring role.

One example of this situation is Ian Murray and his girlfriend. Ian's mother described the girl as 'marvellous - she kept us all together'. She cared for Ian devotedly for three months but then, long before Ian came home, she 'legged it'.

Ian's parents feel that she was under pressure to give him up from her parents. Relationships between the two families had become strained at the hospital, a situation which often seemed to arise in the early weeks (see Chapter One). The girlfriend's mother had taken offence at some remark, and 'from then on it was all downhill'. Ian himself, whose self-confidence had plummeted after the accident, said he is glad that his old girlfriend has left the scene, and none of them ever see her now - 'thank God!' he says. However, Ian was very lonely; he moved away from home and spent all his money on drinking in the evenings. According to his mother, he had difficulty making new friends:

> I think some people sort of see the way he walks, you know he doesn't walk brilliantly...and then his speech is perhaps a little bit slower, and they think, oh I don't want to get to know him, you know. If they try and get to know him then they realize that he's just the same as anybody else.

Three years after his accident, Ian found a new girlfriend, and was intending to get engaged and married. With this relationship some of his self-confidence returned:

> I'm just glad that someone will have me, and I feel all right when I'm with her, she's so much different than my other girlfriend. She understands.

Ian felt that she understood about his problems, and accepted that his arm and his leg did not function properly, because she was also 'slightly disabled'. Ian's father agreed:

> He used to say 'Oh, I'm not going to be no good for nobody,' and he obviously said this to her, you know, 'I'm disabled,' and he calls himself a spastic. And she sort of said to him, 'Ian, the only thing that is wrong with you is that you see yourself as disabled,' she said, 'I don't see that'. She sees through Ian's disabilities and sees Ian for what he is, which I'm very grateful for. He is, underneath, a smashing lad, and a very caring lad.

In spite of Ian's optimism about this relationship, this too came to grief, and Ian is alone again.

Another long-standing relationship that came to grief was that between Ken and his girlfriend. The break-up coincided with the beginning of a period of severe mood swings, but also was the result of Ken's apparent change in attitude towards his girlfriend, a change that his parents found hard to understand:

> She was very good to him up the hospital and until a couple of months ago, and they drifted apart. Now Ken didn't mind that, and yet they'd gone together since school. She was always special to Ken, but when they decided to go their own ways, I think there was partially relief on

Ken's part because she knew his limitations and he prefers people that don't know he's limited.

As with others in the study (see above) Ken finds it easier to mix with people who do not know what he was like before.

Not every relationship comes to grief. Chris Barnes' girlfriend stuck with him, and they are now married, in spite of inter-familial ill-feeling that began at the bedside. Chris's girlfriend stood by him throughout his stay at the hospital, and it is in connection with a telephone call to her that Chris felt that he had made the biggest breakthrough on his road to recovery:

> I phoned up my girlfriend...and I was so proud of myself because I'd remembered her number - at the time my memory was really bad. I couldn't remember one day to the next, and I remembered her phone number, and I suppose it was the first time and the only time I broke down up there. Just something as simple as that just brought it all home. That really did upset me; it seems silly really to pick up the phone and cry, but everyone had been telling me I won't be able to do this, I won't be able to do that, and I did it, all on my own. I remembered that number and I was so chuffed with myself I couldn't speak over the phone...I was really choking.

When he came out of hospital Chris went home to live with his parents for some eighteen months, but he continued to spend a great deal of time with his girlfriend, though usually not on his home ground. To him, she had been the person who had helped him through some of the worst times, even against his will:

> She wouldn't let me sit around moping...she took me up to a pub where I used to go pretty often and it was really scary, I tell you, and everybody, well, some people were really nice, the ones that I knew in there, but it was just really scary. But she pushed me to do it. At the time I held a grudge against her, but she was brilliant.

One other serious relationship also survived. Sylvia Cobb's boyfriend, although he visited her very infrequently in the first few months after the accident, drifted back, and they are considering moving into a house together.

In general, however, it can be seen that few relationships seem to have survived the post head-injury period. For a number of reasons, friends of all sorts from before the accident often seem to drop away. From the friends' point of view, they may find that the young people are significantly changed in personality and interests; they may also be restricted in what they are able, or allowed, to do. From the point of view of the young people themselves, they may well be lacking in confidence, and feel that their friends are patronizing them; they may find the crowded places their friends frequent too threatening; they may not have the same positive feelings as they had for the people with whom they used to spend their time. Thus between them all they let their old friendships atrophy and die. Some may take up with a new set of friends, people who did not know what they were like before the accident, and know them only as they are now. Others stay at home and become socially isolated, remaining dependent on their families for company and support.

they may well be lacking in confidence, and feel that their friends are patronizing them; they may find the crowded places their friends frequent too threatening; they may not have the same positive feelings as they had for the people with whom they used to spend their time. Thus between them all they let their old friendships atrophy and die. Some may take up with a new set of friends, people who did not know what they were like before the accident, and know them only as they are now. Others stay at home and become socially isolated, remaining dependent on their families for company and support.

6 Conclusions

This book has been about the experiences of twenty young people who have suffered a severe head injury, and their families. It has, to a great extent, been written in their own words, and is thus very much their story. There is no doubt that the other people involved - the doctors, nurses, social workers and other professionals, would have given accounts that vary from these, but the specific aim of the research was to document the experience of these families from their own perspectives.

The picture that emerges from their accounts is one of a long and sometimes lonely struggle to try to get back to the lives that they had all led before the accident. There is no preparation for the experience of a severe head injury, either for the people who suffer them or for those who care for them. From the first moments onwards everything that happens is a new, and often traumatic, experience.

The care received in the Accident and Emergency and Intensive Care Units in the various hospitals that people were taken to after their accidents were highly praised by the parents who spent their days and nights at the bedside. Their experiences of subsequent care in hospital, however, were generally unhappy ones, and there were many disturbing accounts of inadequate standards of care on general wards, and a shortage of appropriately trained staff. These complaints about inadequate treatment were made not only about the general wards of small country hospitals, where nursing staff might be expected to have had little experience in the needs of someone recently head injured, but also about the care received in major hospitals in the region.

The families' accounts also demonstrate the inadequacy of the services provided to people once they return home. Parents who take on the task of caring for someone in these circumstances are largely left to cope from day to day in a new and often frightening situation, with little or no advice or support. They are not sure how to treat their head injured children, who often appear to be very different people, and who may behave in strange or violent ways, and lack the insight that they used to have. The tendency is to allow them to take emotional control of the household, by giving in to their demands, and trying to avoid confrontations, in order to keep the peace. Later, parents may come to regret this, but the pattern is set early on, and it is difficult to change direction. When this stage is reached there is usually no one there to turn to, since no professionals are likely to be closely involved with the family by this time. Because no one told them what to expect in the beginning, parents tend to live from day to day, trying to keep the family on an even keel and having to renegotiate their relationship with their unfamiliar son or daughter.

The head injured people have their own, often much more frightening and debilitating problems. They may not always be aware of their own changes in personality, but there is a keen awareness of other changes, such as the loss of skills, of memory problems, lack of confidence and physical effects such as partial paralysis in one arm and leg, deafness, or impaired vision. They may be scared of the nature and extent of their anger and feelings of violence, and unsure of their ability to go into the outside world and function normally among a throng of people who do not know or understand how they feel, who patronise them and label them 'brain-damaged'.

None of these people, those who have been head injured, or their families, could have foreseen the extent of the disruption in their lives, but they could have been much better prepared. Forewarning, advice and continuous support from the beginning might not have eliminated stress and anxiety, but would certainly have alleviated them. Most of these families, once the link with hospital-based professionals is severed, are plunged into limbo. In 1988 Rose wrote that the long-term management of head injured people 'is commonly provided on an *ad hoc* basis and leaves much to be desired, especially in those cases with the greatest need' (Rose 1988: 31). Six years later the situation does not appear to have changed. Even earlier, research showed that a common complaint from relatives of people with a head injury concerned 'poor communication' from professionals (Oddy, Humphrey and Uttley 1978). The situation today seems to be much the same as it was then, some sixteen years ago.

A complicating factor is the nature of the needs that people with a severe head injury, and their families, tend to have. The people described in this book had all made a remarkable recovery from their injury. From a condition in which they were said to be likely to die, or at best remain in a persistent vegetative state, they have, by definition, all recovered enough to live at home. Only Stephie Bell is still unable to walk (apart from a man who also has a spinal injury), and only she and one other have major speech problems. Thus, in general, the people in the study are walking and talking, a few are now working or studying, living as part of a family, out in the 'community'. To the professionals, they may be out of sight and thus out of mind; but for the people themselves, and their families, daily life is beset with problems. There is no doubt that many of the head injured people and their families would benefit from professional input for some years after the accident, but because a parent has taken responsibility for the head injured person, the services seem content to let them get on with it. The needs of the young person, and the families, seldom fit into simple categories, and the parents, by taking their child back, are apparently assumed to be able to cope, whether or not this is so.

In some cases the caring role may continue for years, and in a few cases probably indefinitely. When parents take their son or daughter home from hospital the long term implications are not always considered, and the evidence from this study is that, at a certain point, they would like to get on with their own lives again. 'Informal carers', in the last few years, have developed a high national profile, but their separate needs are not sufficiently considered by the professionals, and it is generally assumed that they will continue in this role, voluntarily, and for as long as necessary, regardless of the personal costs to them. The White Paper 'Caring for People: Community Care in the Next Decade' (Department of Health 1989), and the policy and practice guidelines that have been issued subsequently, acknowledge that carers may have their own separate needs, but they also stress that care managers (and others involved in the assessment of the needs of the person being cared for) should determine what the 'informal sector' can provide before public resources are committed (Parker 1994: 5). Thus, if people with head injury are among those who, in the wake of the NHS and Community Care Act, are to be provided with some sort of care 'package', the parents (or partners) who are currently carrying out a caring role will tend to be incorporated into the care package. This may well reduce the help that is brought in by professionals, and presumably make it less easy for carers to decide not to continue in this role.

The use of the term 'carers' in the context of the aftermath of severe head injury is, in the majority of cases, misleading. Few of the young people would accept that they had a 'carer', and few of the parents would want to be described thus. The role is more a shouldering of responsibility, a caring *about* rather than *for*. It is true that parents in these circumstances will provide shelter and food, but so does one partner for another, without being labelled a 'carer'. The main function of someone who takes responsibility for a person who has had a severe head injury is to watch over and protect them in their current state of vulnerability, to encourage and push gently ahead, and to provide a secure environment from which they can make forays into an outside world that may have been transformed into a confusing and threatening jungle.

Often this protectiveness is carried out in the face of angry resistance, and unreasonable demands. This is partly because parents, in their efforts to protect, may treat their twenty year olds as though they are children again, and from the son or daughter's point of view this is unacceptable. Although it is true that they do become dependent again, for a period at least, and to a greater or lesser extent, this does not mean that it is a childlike dependence. Because most of them were, before the accident, in an interim stage between parental dependence and setting up house with a partner, they all gravitated back to the parental home, at least at first. If they had been older, and established away from home, this would probably not have happened - they would have been treated, by whoever they were with, as an adult who had been injured, instead of being almost forcibly returned to a childhood role.

As the effects of the head injury decrease, it is hard for some parents to let go, whereas others are glad to be able to get on with life as it was before, but for almost all of them the anxiety continues, because they know that the effects of severe head injury will not just disappear, but are likely to continue indefinitely. Some of these parents have already seen their head injured children drift into an empty nomansland, unemployed, without incentive or motivation, and often without hope.

Implications for policy and practice

At a conference held in London in 1993 entitled 'Head Injury Services: Do they work? Are they good enough?' the conclusions were that, after the acute stage, they often do not work, and are certainly not good enough. It was suggested that until 'quite recently' little attention had been given to the 'lengthy process of aftercare and re-integration into the community' (Garrow 1993). However, the fact that little attention has been paid to aftercare services, by those who plan and put into practice head injury rehabilitation programmes, is not through lack of available data, published over the last fifteen years or so, which have clearly indicated the existence of at least some of the social and familial problems that people with head injuries, and their families, encounter in the aftermath of the injury (e.g. Brooks 1984; Lezak 1978; Livingston 1987; Oddy 1984).

The materials presented in this book add a vital perspective to the existing data - that of the people themselves, and their families. The accounts that they give also add considerably to the evidence that head injury services are currently inadequate. If a head injury programme is to be effective from the points of view of all members of the family, there are a number of elements which, according to their own accounts, are absolutely essential.

In hospital:

1 Families should have access to a named member of staff who will provide information about what is happening to their relative in the Accident and Emergency Unit, and in all subsequent in-patient wards. Families should be encouraged to ask questions about any aspects that are of concern to them. General information about the nature of head-injury and the course it may take should also be provided, both verbally and in a simple written form that relatives may keep for reference;

2 Families should receive professional counselling from the beginning, and for as long as necessary, with a counsellor experienced in the problems associated with head injury. At first this would be primarily to help them come to terms with their grief, and later to help each member of the family to adjust to a new situation, and to successfully renegotiate relationships within the family;

3 When the person with a head injury is well enough to be moved out of intensive care, into another ward or hospital, specialist trained staff should be provided to ensure that appropriate treatment continues, to give reassurance, and to answer questions put by members of the family and the head injured person about current procedures and future prospects;

4 The head injured person should be given his or her own professional counsellor (who has specialized knowledge of head injury) as soon as possible in the recovery process.

At home:

5 Counselling should continue for both the person with a head injury, and for members of the family;

6 Rehabilitation should continue as long as needed in any individual case (i.e. not arbitrarily withdrawn), in conjunction with some form of daytime occupation outside the home, whether in a workshop for the

disabled, Headway, or other centre; transport should be provided, however distant from a rehabilitation centre someone may live;

7 The home should be visited regularly by a professional (with specialized knowledge and experience of the effects of severe head injury) whose specific role is to give advice and support to the family, and to assess the nature and extent of the needs of the head injured person and members of the family; this professional should also act as a family 'advocate' to the relevant service authorities, to ensure the provision of appropriate services; he or she should also be easily accessible in emergencies, and to give advice by telephone;

8 As soon as possible, after liaison and negotiation between professionals and employers, the head injured person should be helped to return to paid employment; assistance should also be given to leave the parental home if this is requested, or advisable.

These guidelines are by no means exhaustive, and do not suggest which professionals should take on the various roles, but if these general guidelines were to be followed, the quality of life of people who have suffered severe head injuries, and of their families, would be vastly improved.

Bibliography

Allan, G. A. (1979), *A Sociology of Friendship and Kinship*, Allen & Unwin, London.

Brooks, D. N. (1984), *Closed Head Injury: psychological, social and family consequences*, Oxford University Press, Oxford.

Brooks, D. N. (1991), 'The head-injured family', *Journal of Clinical and Experimental Neuropsychology,* 13, 155-188.

Department of Health (1989), *Caring for People: community care in the next decade,* HMSO, London.

Firth, R., Hubert, J. & Forge A. (1970), *Families and their Relatives,* Routledge & Kegan Paul, London.

Garrow, I. (1993), 'Introduction and welcome of HRH the Princess of Wales', *Head injury services: do they work? Are they good enough?,* Conference Proceedings. St George's Hospital Medical School, London.

Gronwall, D., Wrightson, P. & Waddell P. (1990), *Head Injury: The Facts. A guide for families and care-givers*, Oxford University Press, Oxford.

Lees, M. (1988), 'The social and emotional consequences of severe brain injury: the social work perspective' in Fussey, I. & Giles, G. M. (eds.) *Rehabilitation of the Severely Brain-injured Adult: a practical approach,* Croom Helm, London.

Lezak, M. D. (1978), 'Living with the characterologically altered brain injured patient', *Journal of Clinical Psychiatry,* 39, 592-8.

Livingston, M. G. (1987), 'Head Injury: the relatives' response', *Brain Injury*, 1, 33-39.

Oddy, M. (1984), 'Head injury and social adjustment' in Brooks, N. (ed.), *Closed Head Injury: psychological, social and family consequences*, 108-22. Oxford University Press, Oxford.

Oddy, M., Humphrey, M. & Uttley, D. (1978), 'Stresses upon the relatives of head-injured patients', *British Journal of Psychiatry,* 133, 507-13.

Parker, G. (1994), *Where Next for Research on Carers?,* Nuffield Community Care Studies Unit, Leicester.

Rose, M. (1988), 'Medical considerations in brain injury rehabilitation' in Fussey, I. & Giles, G. M. (eds.) *Rehabilitation of the Severely Brain-injured Adult: a practical approach*, 30-42. Croom Helm, London.

Torrens, M. & Cummins, B. N. n.d. *What is Head Injury*? National Head Injuries Association, London.

Weddell, R., Oddy, M. & Jenkins, D. (1980), 'Social adjustment after rehabilitation: a two year follow-up of patients with severe head injury', *Psychological Medicine,* 10, 257-263.

Note

For further information on head injury (including free pamphlets, booklets and addresses of local Headway Centres) contact Headway (The National Head Injuries Association), 7, King Edward Court, King Edward Street, Nottingham, NG1 1EW (Telephone 01602; Fax 01602 240432).